BREAST CANCER DIET COOKBOOK

FOR WOMEN OVER 50

70 Quick and Easy Nourishing Whole-Food
Transformative Anticancer Recipes for
Prevention and Recovery Featuring Specially
Curated Dishes

ELIZABETH V. CARRINGTON

A SPECIAL THANK YOU

It is with deep gratitude and heartfelt excitement that I welcome you to the pages of "Breast Cancer Diet Cookbook for women over 50." Your choice to explore this nurturing and supportive approach to nutrition during such a crucial time is profoundly appreciated. As a token of my gratitude and to assist you on this new path, I'm offering a personalized service tailored to enhance your experience with this book.

Embarking on a dietary journey following a breast cancer diagnosis can be overwhelming and filled with uncertainties. Whether you're seeking guidance on adapting recipes to your specific nutritional needs, understanding the role of various foods in your recovery, or simply looking for emotional support as you navigate this challenging period, I am here to assist. Consider me not just as an author, but as your personal guide and supporter in this journey.

Please do not hesitate to contact me at elizabethcarringtoncooks@gmail.com with any questions, concerns, or experiences you wish to share. I am dedicated to offering prompt and compassionate responses, ensuring that your journey through this cookbook is not only informative but also comforting and empowering. This is my way of expressing my sincerest thanks and making sure that you have the support you need during this time.

Warm regards,

Elizabeth V. Carrington

TABLE OF CONTENTS

How To Use This Book

1. **Review Recipes**: Skim through the recipes to get an idea of the variety, ingredients used, and the complexity of the dishes. Look for recipes that appeal to your taste preferences and seem manageable given your cooking skills and available time.

2. **Plan Your Meals**: Use the cookbook to plan your weekly meals. Incorporate a variety of recipes to ensure a balanced intake of nutrients. Planning helps make grocery shopping more efficient and reduces food waste.

3. **Make a Shopping List**: Based on your meal plan, create a shopping list. Highlight any ingredients that are new to you or might require a visit to a specialty store. Check your pantry to avoid buying duplicates.

4. **Prep Ingredients**: Some recipes may require prepped ingredients such as washed and

chopped vegetables or marinated proteins. Doing this prep work in advance can save time during cooking.

5. **Cook Recipes**: Start with recipes that seem most appealing and fit your current skill level. Don't be afraid to try new dishes; each recipe is an opportunity to learn something new and enjoy a variety of flavors.

6. **Adjust as Needed**: Feel free to make minor adjustments to the recipes based on your dietary needs and flavor preferences. However, be mindful of substitutions that might alter the nutritional value significantly.

7. **Reflect and Adjust**: After trying a recipe, reflect on what you liked and what you might change next time. Cooking is a personal and evolving process, and it's okay to tweak

recipes to better suit your tastes and nutritional needs.

APPETIZERS

RECIPE 1

ROASTED RED PEPPER AND WALNUT DIP

Serves: 6-8 | Prep Time: 15 minutes | Cooking Time: 15 minutes | Total Time: 30 minutes

Ingredients:

- 2 large red bell peppers

- 1/2 cup walnuts, toasted

- 2 cloves garlic, minced

- 2 tablespoons olive oil

- 1 tablespoon lemon juice

- 1 teaspoon ground cumin

- 1/2 teaspoon paprika

- Salt and pepper to taste

- Fresh parsley leaves for garnish (optional)

Instructions:

1. Set your oven to 450°F (230°C).

2. Place the whole red bell peppers directly on the oven rack or a baking sheet lined with aluminum foil. Roast the peppers for about 15-20 minutes, turning them occasionally until the skin is charred and blistered.

3. Remove the peppers from the oven and immediately transfer them to a bowl. Cover the bowl with plastic wrap or a lid and let the peppers steam for about 10 minutes. This helps the skin to peel off easily.

4. Once the peppers have cooled a bit, peel off the skin, remove the seeds, and chop them into

smaller pieces.

5. In a food processor, combine the roasted red peppers, toasted walnuts, minced garlic, olive oil, lemon juice, ground cumin, paprika, salt, and pepper.

6. Process the mixture until smooth and creamy. You may need to scrape down the sides of the food processor a few times to ensure everything is well blended.

7. Taste the dip and adjust the seasoning if needed. You can add more lemon juice, cumin, salt, or pepper according to your preference.

8. Transfer the dip to a serving bowl, garnish with fresh parsley leaves if desired, and serve with your favorite dipping accompaniments, such as pita bread, crackers, or vegetable sticks.

Nutritional Information (Per Serving - 1/8th of the recipe):

Calories: 115| Total Fat: 11g| Saturated Fat: 1g| Cholesterol: 0mg| Sodium: 118mg| Total Carbohydrates: 4g| Dietary Fiber: 1g| Sugars: 1g| Protein: 2g

RECIPE 2

CUCUMBER AND HUMMUS BITES

Serves: 4-6| Prep Time: 15 minutes| Cooking Time: None| Total Time: 15 minutes

Ingredients:

- 2 large cucumbers

- 1 cup hummus (store-bought or homemade)

- Cherry tomatoes, for garnish

- Fresh parsley or dill leaves, for garnish (optional)

- Olive oil, for drizzling (optional)

- Salt and pepper to taste

Instructions:

1. Wash and peel the cucumbers (you can leave some strips of skin for a decorative touch). Slice the cucumbers into rounds, about 1/2-inch thick.

2. Use a small spoon or melon baller to scoop out a small indentation in the center of each cucumber round. This will create a small well to hold the hummus.

3. Fill each cucumber well with a spoonful of hummus. You can also use a piping bag or plastic bag with a corner cut off to pipe the hummus neatly into the cucumbers.

4. Garnish each cucumber and hummus bite with a small cherry tomato half. If desired, you can also add a small leaf of fresh parsley or dill on top for extra flavor and presentation.

5. Season the bites with a pinch of salt and pepper to taste.

6. Optional: Drizzle a bit of olive oil over the top for added richness (this step is entirely optional).

7. Arrange the cucumber and hummus bites on a serving platter, and they are ready to be enjoyed as a healthy and refreshing appetizer.

Nutritional Information (Per Serving - 2 cucumber and hummus bites):

Calories: 84| Total Fat: 4g| Saturated Fat: 1g|

Cholesterol: 0mg| Sodium: 245mg| Total Carbohydrates: 10g| Dietary Fiber: 2g| Sugars: 2g| Protein: 3g

RECIPE 3

ZUCCHINI AND CARROT FRITTERS

Serves: 4| Prep Time: 20 minutes| Cooking Time: 15 minutes| Total Time: 35 minutes

Ingredients:

- 2 medium zucchinis, grated

- 2 medium carrots, grated

- 1/2 cup breadcrumbs (preferably whole wheat)

- 1/4 cup grated Parmesan cheese (optional)

- 2 cloves garlic, minced and 2 large eggs, beaten

- 2 tablespoons fresh parsley, chopped

- 1/2 teaspoon salt, or to taste

- 1/4 teaspoon black pepper, or to taste

- Olive oil for frying

Instructions:

1. Grate the zucchinis and carrots using a box grater. Place them in a clean kitchen towel or cheesecloth, and squeeze out as much liquid as possible. This step is important to prevent soggy fritters.

2. In a large mixing bowl, combine the grated zucchinis and carrots, breadcrumbs, Parmesan cheese (if using), minced garlic, beaten eggs, chopped fresh parsley, salt, and black pepper. Mix everything together until well combined.

3. Heat a non-stick skillet or frying pan over medium heat and add enough olive oil to coat the bottom of the pan.

4. Once the oil is hot, use a spoon to drop portions of the mixture into the pan, flattening them slightly with the back of the spoon to form fritters.

5. Cook the fritters for about 3-4 minutes on each side, or until they are golden brown and crispy. Depending on how large your pan is, you may need to work in batches.

6. Place cooked fritters on a paper towel-lined plate to drain any excess oil.

7. Serve the zucchini and carrot fritters hot, garnished with additional fresh parsley if desired.

Nutritional Information (Per Serving - 1/4 of the recipe):

Calories: 189| Total Fat: 9g| Saturated Fat: 2g| Cholesterol: 98mg| Sodium: 452mg| Total Carbohydrates: 19g| Dietary Fiber: 3g| Sugars: 4g| Protein: 8g

RECIPE 4

BAKED KALE CHIPS WITH NUTRITIONAL YEAST

Serves: 2-4| Prep Time: 10 minutes| Cooking Time: 12-15 minutes| Total Time: 22-25 minutes

Ingredients:

- 1 bunch of fresh kale

- 2 tablespoons olive oil

- 2 tablespoons nutritional yeast

- Salt and pepper to taste

Instructions:

1. Set your oven to 350°F (175°C).

2. Give the kale leaves a good wash and let them air dry. You may wipe them dry with a fresh kitchen towel or use a salad spinner.

3. Remove the tough stems from the kale leaves, as they can be bitter. Tear the kale into bite-sized pieces.

4. In a large mixing bowl, drizzle the olive oil over the kale leaves. Make sure the leaves are uniformly covered by massaging the oil into them with your hands.

5. Sprinkle nutritional yeast over the kale leaves. Nutritional yeast adds a cheesy flavor and is rich in B vitamins. Toss the kale to distribute the

nutritional yeast evenly.

6. Season the kale chips with a pinch of salt and a dash of pepper according to your taste. Be cautious with the salt, as nutritional yeast can be salty as well.

7. Line a baking sheet with parchment paper. Spread out the kale leaves in a single layer on the baking sheet.

8. Bake the kale chips in the preheated oven for 12-15 minutes, or until they are crisp and the edges are slightly browned. Keep a close eye on them to prevent burning.

9. Remove the kale chips from the oven and let them cool for a few minutes.

10. Transfer the baked kale chips to a serving bowl or plate, and they are ready to be enjoyed as a healthy and flavorful snack.

Nutritional Information (Per Serving - 1/4 of the recipe):

Calories: 80| Total Fat: 60| Saturated Fat: 1g| Cholesterol: 0mg| Sodium: 50mg| Total Carbohydrates: 5g| Dietary Fiber: 1g| Sugars: 0g| Protein: 3g

RECIPE 5

TOMATO AND BASIL BRUSCHETTA ON WHOLE GRAIN BREAD

Serves: 4| Prep Time: 15 minutes| Cooking Time: 5 minutes| Total Time: 20 minutes

Ingredients:

- 4 slices of whole grain bread

- 4 ripe tomatoes, diced

- 2 cloves garlic, minced

- 1/4 cup fresh basil leaves, chopped

- 2 tablespoons extra-virgin olive oil

- 1 teaspoon balsamic vinegar (optional)

- Salt and pepper to taste

Instructions:

1. Preheat your oven's broiler or a toaster oven to medium-high heat.

2. Place the slices of whole grain bread on a baking sheet and toast them under the broiler or in the toaster oven until they are golden brown. Don't take your eyes off them to avoid getting them burned. This should take about 3-5 minutes.

3. In a mixing bowl, combine the diced tomatoes,

minced garlic, chopped fresh basil, extra-virgin olive oil, and balsamic vinegar (if using). Toss everything together until well combined.

4. Season the tomato and basil mixture with a pinch of salt and pepper to taste. Be cautious with the salt, as the bread will also contribute some saltiness.

5. Once the bread slices are toasted, remove them from the oven and let them cool slightly.

6. Spoon the tomato and basil mixture generously onto each slice of toasted bread, spreading it evenly.

7. Serve the Tomato and Basil Bruschetta immediately as a delicious appetizer or snack.

Nutritional Information (Per Serving - 1 slice of bruschetta):

Calories: 182| Total Fat: 9g| Saturated Fat: 1g| Cholesterol: 0mg| Sodium: 220mg| Total Carbohydrates: 21g| Dietary Fiber: 4g| Sugars: 4g| Protein: 4g

RECIPE 6

AVOCADO AND SHRIMP COCKTAIL CUPS

Serves: 4| Prep Time: 20 minutes| Cooking Time: 5 minutes| Total Time: 25 minutes

Ingredients:

For the Shrimp:

- 1/2 pound large shrimp, peeled and deveined

- 1 lemon, cut into wedges

- Salt and pepper to taste

For the Cocktail Sauce:

- 1/2 cup ketchup

- 2 tablespoons prepared horseradish

- 1 tablespoon lemon juice

- 1 teaspoon Worcestershire sauce

- A few dashes of hot sauce (adjust to your spice preference)

For the Avocado Cups:

- 1 tablespoon lemon juice (for brushing the avocados)

- Fresh parsley or cilantro leaves for garnish

(optional)

- 2 ripe avocados

Instructions:

1. Prepare the Shrimp: - Bring a saucepan of water to a boil. Add the shrimp and simmer for approximately 2-3 minutes, or until they become pink and opaque.

  - Drain the shrimp and immediately transfer them to a dish of cold water to halt the frying process. Once cooled, drain again.

  - Squeeze lemon juice over the cooked shrimp and season with salt and pepper. Set aside.

2. Prepare the Cocktail Sauce: - In a small bowl, whisk together ketchup, prepared horseradish, lemon juice, Worcestershire sauce, and spicy sauce. Adjust the spicy sauce to your preferred degree of heat. Refrigerate the sauce until ready to use.

3. Prepare the Avocado Cups: - Cut the avocados in half lengthwise and remove the seeds.

- Brush the cut sides of the avocados with lemon juice to avoid browning.

4. Assemble the Avocado and Shrimp Cocktail Cups: - Place a teaspoon of cocktail sauce into each avocado half.

- Arrange the cooked shrimp on top of the cocktail sauce in each avocado half.

- Garnish with fresh parsley or cilantro leaves if preferred.

5. Serve the Avocado and Shrimp Cocktail Cups immediately as an exquisite appetizer or starter.

Nutritional Information (Per Serving - 1/4 of the recipe):

Calories: 242| Total Fat: 12g| Saturated Fat:

2g| Cholesterol: 105mg| Sodium: 707mg| Total Carbohydrates: 21g| Dietary Fiber: 6g| Sugars: 11g| Protein: 14g

RECIPE 7

SPINACH AND FETA STUFFED MUSHROOMS

Serves: 4| Prep Time: 15 minutes| Cooking Time: 20 minutes| Total Time: 35 minutes

Ingredients:

- 12 large button mushrooms

- 2 cups fresh spinach, finely chopped

- 1/2 cup crumbled feta cheese

- 2 cloves garlic, minced

- 2 tablespoons olive oil

- 1/4 cup breadcrumbs (preferably whole wheat)

- Salt and pepper to taste

- Fresh parsley leaves for garnish (optional)

Instructions:

1. Set your oven to 375°F (190°C).

2. Clean the mushrooms by wiping them with a damp cloth or paper towel. Remove the stems and set them aside.

3. In a pan, heat olive oil over medium heat.

Add minced garlic and sauté for approximately 1 minute until fragrant.

4. Add the chopped spinach to the skillet and sauté for another 2-3 minutes until it wilts and any excess moisture evaporates. Season with salt and pepper to taste.

5. In a mixing bowl, combine the cooked spinach, crumbled feta cheese, and breadcrumbs. Mix everything together until well combined.

6. Take each mushroom cap and stuff it with the spinach and feta mixture, pressing down gently to pack the filling.

7. Arrange the filled mushrooms on a baking sheet lined with parchment paper.

8. Bake the stuffed mushrooms in the preheated oven for about 15-20 minutes, or until the

mushrooms are tender and the filling is golden brown.

9. Once cooked, remove the stuffed mushrooms from the oven and let them cool slightly.

10. Garnish with fresh parsley leaves if desired, and serve the Spinach and Feta Stuffed Mushrooms as a delightful appetizer.

Nutritional Information (Per Serving - 1/4 of the recipe):

Calories: 133| Total Fat: 9g| Saturated Fat: 3g| Cholesterol: 11mg| Sodium: 237mg| Total Carbohydrates: 8g| Dietary Fiber: 1g| Sugars: 1g| Protein: 5g

RECIPE 8

SWEET POTATO AND BLACK BEAN MINI TACOS

Serves: 4 | Prep Time: 15 minutes | Cooking Time: 25 minutes | Total Time: 40 minutes

Ingredients:

For the Sweet Potato Filling:

- 2 medium sweet potatoes, peeled and diced into small cubes

- 1 tablespoon olive oil

- 1 teaspoon chili powder

- 1/2 teaspoon cumin

- Salt and pepper to taste

For the Black Bean Topping:

- 1 can (15 oz) black beans, drained and rinsed

- 1/2 teaspoon garlic powder

- 1/2 teaspoon onion powder

- Salt and pepper to taste

For Assembling:

- Mini taco shells or tortillas

- Sliced avocado

- Salsa

- Fresh cilantro leaves for garnish (optional)

- Lime wedges for serving (optional)

Instructions:

1. Set your oven to 425°F (220°C).

2. In a large mixing bowl, toss the diced sweet potatoes with olive oil, chili powder, cumin, salt, and pepper until they are evenly coated.

3. Spread the seasoned sweet potatoes on a baking sheet in a single layer. Roast them in the preheated oven for about 20-25 minutes or until they are tender and slightly crispy, turning them halfway through the cooking time.

4. While the sweet potatoes are roasting, prepare the black bean topping. In a saucepan, heat the drained and rinsed black beans over medium heat. Add onion powder, garlic powder, pepper, and salt. Cook for about 5 minutes, stirring occasionally, until heated through and well-seasoned.

5. Warm the mini taco shells or tortillas according to the package instructions.

6. To assemble the mini tacos, fill each taco shell with a spoonful of roasted sweet potatoes, a portion of black beans, sliced avocado, salsa, and garnish with fresh cilantro leaves if desired.

7. Serve the Sweet Potato and Black Bean Mini Tacos with lime wedges for an optional citrusy kick.

Nutritional Information (Per Serving - 1/4 of the recipe, without optional garnishes):

Calories: 230| Total Fat: 5g| Saturated Fat: 1g| Cholesterol: 0mg| Sodium: 405mg| Total Carbohydrates: 41g| Dietary Fiber: 10g| Sugars: 6g| Protein: 7g

RECIPE 9

EDAMAME AND MINT DIP WITH WHOLE WHEAT PITA CHIPS

Serves: 4| Prep Time: 15 minutes| Cooking Time: 10 minutes (for pita chips)| Total Time: 25 minutes

Ingredients:

For the Edamame and Mint Dip:

- 1 1/2 cups shelled edamame (frozen or fresh)

- 2 cloves garlic, minced

- 1/4 cup fresh mint leaves

- 2 tablespoons fresh lemon juice

- 2 tablespoons tahini

- 2 tablespoons extra-virgin olive oil

- Salt and pepper to taste

- Water (for adjusting consistency)

For the Whole Wheat Pita Chips:

- 2 whole wheat pita breads, cut into triangles

- 1 tablespoon olive oil

- 1/2 teaspoon paprika

- 1/4 teaspoon garlic powder

- Salt to taste

Instructions:

1. Prepare the Edamame and Mint Dip:

   - Get information from the package instructions on how to cook the shelled edamame. Drain and let them cool slightly.

- In a food processor, combine the cooked edamame, minced garlic, fresh mint leaves, fresh lemon juice, tahini, and extra-virgin olive oil.

- Blend until the mixture becomes smooth. If the dip is too thick, you can add a little water to reach your desired consistency.

- Add salt and pepper to your desired taste. Adjust the seasonings as needed.

2. Prepare the Whole Wheat Pita Chips:

- Set your oven to 350°F (175°C).

- Cut the whole wheat pita breads into triangles or desired chip shapes.

- In a bowl, toss the pita triangles with olive oil, paprika, garlic powder, and a pinch of salt until they are well coated.

- Arrange the seasoned pita triangles on a

baking sheet in a single layer.

- Bake in the preheated oven for about 8-10 minutes or until the pita chips are crisp and lightly browned. Keep a proper check on them to avoid burning

3. Serve the Edamame and Mint Dip with the Whole Wheat Pita Chips as a healthy and flavorful snack or appetizer.

Nutritional Information (Per Serving - 1/4 of the recipe, without optional garnishes):

Calories: 250| Total Fat: 14g| Saturated Fat: 2g| Cholesterol: 0mg| Sodium: 230mg| Total Carbohydrates: 22g| Dietary Fiber: 6g| Sugars: 2g| Protein: 9g

RECIPE 10

GRILLED ASPARAGUS SPEARS WRAPPED IN PROSCIUTTO

Serves: 4 | Prep Time: 15 minutes | Cooking Time: 10 minutes | Total Time: 25 minutes

Ingredients:

- 1 bunch of fresh asparagus spears (about 16 spears)

- 8 slices of prosciutto

- 2 tablespoons extra-virgin olive oil

- Freshly ground black pepper, to taste

- Balsamic reduction (optional, for drizzling)

Instructions:

1. Preheat your grill to medium-high heat.

2. Wash the asparagus spears and trim off the tough ends. You can do this by snapping off the woody ends at the natural breaking point.

3. Divide the asparagus spears into 8 equal portions, as you'll be wrapping each portion with a slice of prosciutto.

4. Take a slice of prosciutto and lay it flat on a clean surface. Place a portion of asparagus spears at one end of the prosciutto slice.

5. Carefully roll the prosciutto around the asparagus, making sure it wraps snugly.

6. Repeat the process for all asparagus portions.

7. Drizzle the wrapped asparagus spears with extra-virgin olive oil and season them with freshly ground black pepper.

8. Place the wrapped asparagus on the preheated grill. Grill for about 2-3 minutes per side, or until the prosciutto is crispy and the

asparagus is tender-crisp.

9. Remove the grilled asparagus spears from the grill and arrange them on a serving platter.

10. Optional: Drizzle with balsamic reduction for added flavor.

11. Serve the Grilled Asparagus Spears Wrapped in Prosciutto as a delicious appetizer or side dish.

Nutritional Information (Per Serving - 1/4 of the recipe):

Calories: 80| Total Fat: 5g| Saturated Fat: 1g| Cholesterol: 15mg| Sodium: 390mg| Total Carbohydrates: 2g| Dietary Fiber: 1g| Sugars: 1g| Protein: 6g

Breakfast Recipes

Recipe 1

Avocado and Egg Toast on Whole Grain Bread

Serves: 1 serving| Prep Time: 5 minutes| Cooking Time: 5 minutes| Total Time: 10 minutes

Ingredients:

- 1 slice of whole grain bread

- 1/2 ripe avocado

- 1 egg

- Salt and pepper, to taste

- Optional toppings: red pepper flakes, fresh herbs (such as cilantro or parsley), or a squeeze of lemon juice

Instructions:

1. Toast the Bread: Place the whole grain bread in a toaster and toast it to your preferred level of crispiness.

2. Cook the Egg: While the bread is toasting, cook the egg to your liking. You can either fry, poach, or soft boil the egg. For a fried egg, heat a non-stick skillet over medium heat, crack the egg into the pan, and cook until the whites are set and the yolk is still slightly runny, or fully cooked if that's your preference. Add a little salt and pepper.

3. Prepare the Avocado: Cut the avocado in half and remove the pit. Scoop out the flesh of one half and use a fork to mash it in a small bowl. You can season the mashed avocado with a little salt, pepper, and optional lemon juice for extra flavor.

4. Assemble the Toast: Spread the mashed avocado evenly over the toasted bread. Get the cooked egg and place on top of the avocado carefully.

5. Add Final Touches: Season the avocado and egg toast with additional salt and pepper to taste. If desired, sprinkle some red pepper flakes or fresh herbs on top for an extra flavor kick.

6. Serve: Enjoy your avocado and egg toast immediately while it's still warm.

Nutritional Information (per serving, approximate):

Calories: 300 kcal| Protein: 12 g| Fat: 20 g (Saturated: 4 g, Unsaturated: 14 g)| Carbohydrates: 20 g (Fiber: 7 g, Sugars: 3 g)| Cholesterol: 185 mg| Sodium: 400 mg

RECIPE 2

GREEK YOGURT PARFAIT WITH MIXED BERRIES AND ALMONDS

Serves: 2 servings | Prep Time: 10 minutes | Cooking Time: 0 minutes (no cooking required) | Total Time: 10 minutes

Ingredients:

- 1 cup Greek yogurt (plain or vanilla)

- 1/2 cup mixed berries (such as strawberries, blueberries, raspberries, and blackberries), fresh or frozen and thawed

- 1/4 cup granola

- 2 tablespoons almonds, sliced or chopped

- 1 tablespoon honey or maple syrup (optional)

- A few mint leaves for garnish (optional)

Instructions:

1. Prepare the Berries: If using fresh berries, wash them thoroughly and pat dry. If using frozen berries, ensure they are thawed completely. Slice any larger berries like strawberries into smaller pieces for easier eating.

2. Layer the Parfait: Begin assembling the parfait by spooning a layer of Greek yogurt at the bottom of two glasses or parfait dishes. Follow this with a layer of mixed berries.

3. Add Crunch: Sprinkle a layer of granola over the berries, and then add a few sliced almonds for an extra crunch.

4. Repeat Layers: Repeat the layers until the glasses are filled to the top, finishing with a layer of berries and almonds.

5. Sweeten (Optional): Drizzle a little honey or

maple syrup over the top for added sweetness, if desired.

6. Garnish and Serve: Garnish with mint leaves for a fresh touch and an extra pop of color. You can refrigerate or serve without wasting time.

Nutritional Information (per serving, approximate):

Calories: 220 kcal| Protein: 12 g| Fat: 8 g (Saturated: 1 g, Unsaturated: 7 g)| Carbohydrates: 28 g (Fiber: 4 g, Sugars: 18 g)| Cholesterol: 5 mg| Sodium: 50 mg

RECIPE 3

OATMEAL WITH SLICED APPLE, CINNAMON, AND WALNUTS

Serves: 2 servings| Prep Time: 5 minutes| Cooking Time: 10 minutes| Total Time: 15 minutes

Ingredients:

- 1 cup rolled oats

- 2 cups water or milk (for creamier oatmeal, use milk)

- 1 medium apple, cored and thinly sliced

- 1/2 teaspoon ground cinnamon

- 2 tablespoons walnuts, chopped

- 1 tablespoon honey or maple syrup (optional)

- Pinch of salt

Instructions:

1. Cook the Oats: In a medium saucepan, bring the water or milk to a boil. Add a pinch of salt and stir in the rolled oats. Reduce the heat to a simmer and cook, stirring occasionally, for about 5 minutes or until the oats are soft and have absorbed most of the liquid.

2. Add Flavors: Halfway through cooking, add the ground cinnamon and half of the sliced apples to the oatmeal, stirring them in. This allows the apples to soften slightly and infuses the oatmeal with their flavor.

3. Serve: Once the oatmeal is cooked to your desired consistency, remove it from the heat. Spoon the oatmeal into two bowls.

4. Garnish and Sweeten: Top each bowl with the remaining apple slices, chopped walnuts, and a drizzle of honey or maple syrup if a sweeter taste is desired.

5. Serve Hot: Enjoy your oatmeal hot for a comforting and nutritious meal.

Nutritional Information (per serving, approximate):

Calories: 300 kcal| Protein: 8 g| Fat: 10 g (Saturated: 1 g, Unsaturated: 9 g)| Carbohydrates: 50 g (Fiber: 7 g, Sugars: 15 g)| Cholesterol: 0 mg| Sodium: 30 mg

RECIPE 4

SMOOTHIE BOWL WITH SPINACH, BANANA, AND FLAXSEEDS, TOPPED WITH PUMPKIN SEEDS

Serves: 1 serving| Prep Time: 10 minutes|
Cooking Time: 0 minutes (no cooking required) |
Total Time: 10 minutes

Ingredients:

- 1 large ripe banana, frozen and sliced

- 1 cup fresh spinach leaves, washed

- 1 tablespoon flaxseeds

- 1/2 cup unsweetened almond milk (or any milk
of your choice)

- 1/4 cup Greek yogurt (for added creaminess,
optional)

- Toppings:

  - 1 tablespoon pumpkin seeds

  - Additional banana slices (optional)

  - A few berries (optional)

- A sprinkle of chia seeds (optional)

Instructions:

1. Blend the Smoothie: In a high-speed blender, combine the frozen banana slices, fresh spinach leaves, flaxseeds, almond milk, and Greek yogurt (if using). The mixture should be smooth and creamy after blending on high. If additional almond milk is required, adjust the consistency.

2. Prepare the Bowl: Pour the smoothie mixture into a bowl.

3. Add Toppings: Sprinkle pumpkin seeds over the top of the smoothie bowl. If desired, add additional banana slices, a handful of berries, and a sprinkle of chia seeds for extra nutrition and flavor.

4. Serve Immediately: Enjoy your smoothie bowl immediately for the best texture and taste.

Nutritional Information (per serving, approximate):

Calories: 330 kcal| Protein: 10 g| Fat: 10 g (Saturated: 1 g, Unsaturated: 9 g)| Carbohydrates: 53 g (Fiber: 9 g, Sugars: 25 g) | Cholesterol: 0 mg| Sodium: 150 mg

RECIPE 5

COTTAGE CHEESE WITH PINEAPPLE CHUNKS AND A SPRINKLE OF CHIA SEEDS

Serves: 1 serving| Prep Time: 5 minutes| Cooking Time: 0 minutes (no cooking required) | Total Time: 5 minutes

Ingredients:

- 1 cup low-fat cottage cheese

- 1/2 cup pineapple chunks (fresh or canned in juice, drained)

- 1 tablespoon chia seeds

Instructions:

1. Prepare the Ingredients: If you're using fresh pineapple, peel, core, and cut it into small chunks. If you're using canned pineapple, ensure it's drained well to remove excess juice.

2. Assemble the Dish: In a serving bowl, place the cottage cheese as the base layer.

3. Add Pineapple: Distribute the pineapple chunks evenly over the cottage cheese.

4. Sprinkle Chia Seeds: Sprinkle the chia seeds

over the top of the pineapple and cottage cheese.

5. Serve: Enjoy immediately as a refreshing and nutritious breakfast, snack, or dessert.

Nutritional Information (per serving, approximate):

Calories: 250 kcal| Protein: 28 g| Fat: 5 g (Saturated: 1 g, Unsaturated: 4 g)| Carbohydrates: 20 g (Fiber: 5 g, Sugars: 15 g) | Cholesterol: 10 mg| Sodium: 500 mg

RECIPE 6

BUCKWHEAT PANCAKES WITH BLUEBERRY COMPOTE

Serves: 4 servings | Prep Time: 15 minutes | Cooking Time: 20 minutes | Total Time: 35 minutes

Ingredients:

For the Pancakes:

- 1 cup buckwheat flour

- 1 tablespoon sugar (optional)

- 1 teaspoon baking powder

- 1/2 teaspoon baking soda

- 1/4 teaspoon salt

- 1 1/4 cups buttermilk (or a mixture of milk and a tablespoon of lemon juice or vinegar)

- 1 large egg

- 2 tablespoons unsalted butter, melted, plus more for cooking

For the Blueberry Compote:

- 2 cups fresh or frozen blueberries

- 1/4 cup water

- 2 tablespoons sugar, or to taste

- 1 teaspoon lemon juice

Instructions:

1. Make the Blueberry Compote: In a small saucepan, combine blueberries, water, sugar, and lemon juice. While stirring occasionally, bring to a simmer over medium heat. Cook until the berries have burst and the sauce has thickened slightly, about 10 minutes. Remove from heat and set aside to cool.

2. Prepare the Pancake Batter: In a large bowl,

whisk together buckwheat flour, sugar (if using), baking powder, baking soda, and salt. In another bowl, beat the egg with the buttermilk and melted butter. Pour the wet ingredients into the dry ingredients, stirring until just combined. Be careful not to overmix.

3. Cook the Pancakes: Heat a non-stick skillet or griddle over medium heat and brush with a little melted butter. Pour about 1/4 cup of batter for each pancake onto the skillet. Cook until bubbles form on the surface and the edges look set, about 2 minutes. Flip the pancakes and cook until the other side is golden brown, about 1-2 more minutes. Repeat this process with the remaining batter, then add more butter to the skillet as required.

4. Serve: Serve the pancakes warm, topped with the blueberry compote.

Nutritional Information (per serving, approximate):

Calories: 350 kcal| Protein: 8 g| Fat: 10 g (Saturated: 5 g, Unsaturated: 5 g)| Carbohydrates: 58 g (Fiber: 5 g, Sugars: 24 g) | Cholesterol: 65 mg| Sodium: 500 mg

RECIPE 7

QUINOA PORRIDGE WITH ALMOND MILK AND DRIED APRICOTS

Serves: 2 servings| Prep Time: 5 minutes| Cooking Time: 20 minutes| Total Time: 25 minutes

Ingredients:

- 1/2 cup quinoa, rinsed and drained

- 2 cups unsweetened almond milk, plus more

for serving

- 1/4 cup dried apricots, chopped

- 1 tablespoon honey or maple syrup, plus more for serving

- 1/2 teaspoon cinnamon

- Pinch of salt

- Optional toppings: sliced almonds, chia seeds, additional chopped apricots, a sprinkle of cinnamon

Instructions:

1. Cook Quinoa: In a medium saucepan, combine the rinsed quinoa, almond milk, cinnamon, and a pinch of salt. Bring the mixture to a boil over medium-high heat.

2. Simmer: Once boiling, reduce the heat to low,

cover, and simmer for 15-20 minutes, or until the quinoa is tender and has absorbed most of the almond milk.

3. Add Apricots: Stir in the chopped dried apricots and honey or maple syrup into the cooked quinoa. Cook for an additional 2-3 minutes, or until the apricots have softened slightly.

4. Serve: Divide the porridge between two bowls. If the porridge is too thick, you can add a little more almond milk to reach your desired consistency.

5. Add Toppings: Garnish with your choice of toppings such as sliced almonds, chia seeds, additional chopped apricots, or a sprinkle of cinnamon.

6. Enjoy: Serve warm with an extra drizzle of honey or maple syrup, if desired.

Nutritional Information (per serving, approximate):

Calories: 250 kcal| Protein: 6 g| Fat: 5 g (Saturated: 0 g, Unsaturated: 5 g)| Carbohydrates: 45 g (Fiber: 5 g, Sugars: 15 g) | Cholesterol: 0 mg| Sodium: 100 mg

RECIPE 8

SCRAMBLED TOFU WITH KALE AND TOMATOES

Serves: 2 servings| Prep Time: 10 minutes| Cooking Time: 10 minutes| Total Time: 20 minutes

Ingredients:

- 1 block (14 oz) firm tofu, drained and crumbled

- 2 cups kale, washed and roughly chopped

- 1 medium tomato, diced

- 1/2 onion, finely chopped

- 2 cloves garlic, minced

- 1/4 teaspoon turmeric (for color)

- Salt and pepper, to taste

- 1 tablespoon olive oil

- Optional: 1/4 teaspoon smoked paprika or cumin for extra flavor

- Optional garnish: chopped fresh herbs (such as parsley or cilantro), avocado slices

Instructions:

1. Prepare the Ingredients: Drain the tofu and press it between paper towels to remove excess moisture. Crumble the tofu into small pieces. Wash and chop the kale, dice the tomato, and finely chop the onion and garlic.

2. Cook the Onion and Garlic: Heat the olive oil in a large skillet over medium heat. Add the onion and garlic, sautéing until the onion is translucent and fragrant, about 2-3 minutes.

3. Add Tofu and Spices: Add the crumbled tofu to the skillet along with turmeric, salt, pepper, and any additional spices you're using. Cook for 5-7 minutes, stirring occasionally, until the tofu is heated through and starting to get a bit golden.

4. Incorporate Kale and Tomatoes: Add the chopped kale and diced tomatoes to the skillet. Cook for an additional 3-5 minutes, or until the kale has wilted and the tomatoes are warmed through.

5. Final Seasoning: Taste and adjust the seasoning with more salt and pepper if needed.

6. Serve: Divide the scrambled tofu mixture between two plates. Garnish with fresh herbs or avocado slices if desired.

Nutritional Information (per serving, approximate):

Calories: 250 kcal| Protein: 18 g| Fat: 15 g (Saturated: 2 g, Unsaturated: 13 g)| Carbohydrates: 15 g (Fiber: 4 g, Sugars: 4 g)| Cholesterol: 0 mg| Sodium: 200 mg

RECIPE 9

MUESLI WITH SKIMMED MILK, SLICED PEAR, AND SUNFLOWER SEEDS

Serves: 1 serving| Prep Time: 5 minutes| Cooking Time: 0 minutes (no cooking required)| Total Time: 5 minutes

Ingredients:

- 1/2 cup muesli

- 3/4 cup skimmed milk

- 1 medium pear, cored and thinly sliced

- 1 tablespoon sunflower seeds

Instructions:

1. Prepare the Ingredients: Core the pear and cut it into thin slices. Measure out the muesli and sunflower seeds.

2. Assemble the Muesli: In a serving bowl, combine the muesli with the skimmed milk. Stir to mix well.

3. Add the Pear: Arrange the sliced pear on top of the muesli.

4. Garnish with Sunflower Seeds: Sprinkle the

sunflower seeds over the pear.

5. Serve: Enjoy your bowl of muesli immediately, or let it sit for a few minutes if you prefer the muesli to soften slightly in the milk.

Nutritional Information (per serving, approximate):

Calories: 350 kcal| Protein: 12 g| Fat: 5 g (Saturated: 0.5 g, Unsaturated: 4.5 g) | Carbohydrates: 65 g (Fiber: 9 g, Sugars: 25 g) | Cholesterol: 2 mg| Sodium: 100 mg

RECIPE 10

Baked Sweet Potato and Black Bean Breakfast Burritos

Serves: 4 servings| Prep Time: 15 minutes| Cooking Time: 25 minutes for sweet potatoes +

10 minutes for burritos | Total Time: 50 minutes

Ingredients:

- 2 medium sweet potatoes, peeled and diced

- 1 tablespoon olive oil

- 1 teaspoon ground cumin

- Salt and pepper, to taste

- 1 cup canned black beans, drained and rinsed

- 4 large whole wheat tortillas

- 4 eggs, lightly beaten

- 1/2 cup shredded cheese (cheddar or Monterey Jack)

- Optional garnishes: avocado slices, salsa, sour cream, cilantro

Instructions:

1. Preheat Oven and Prepare Sweet Potatoes
Preheat the oven to 400°F (200°C). Toss the diced sweet potatoes with olive oil, cumin, salt, and pepper on a baking sheet. Spread them out in a single layer. Bake for about 25 minutes or until tender and lightly browned, stirring halfway through.

2. Scramble the Eggs: While the sweet potatoes are baking, heat a non-stick skillet over medium heat. Add the beaten eggs and scramble until they are just set. Season with salt and pepper to taste. Set aside.

3. Assemble the Burritos: Lay out the whole wheat tortillas on a flat surface. Divide the roasted sweet potato, scrambled eggs, black beans, and shredded cheese evenly among the tortillas. Fold in the sides of each tortilla and roll up tightly to form the burritos.

4. Bake the Burritos: Place the assembled

burritos seam side down on a baking sheet. Bake in the preheated oven for about 10 minutes, or until the tortillas are crispy and the cheese has melted.

5. Serve: Serve the baked burritos hot with optional garnishes like avocado slices, salsa, sour cream, or cilantro.

Nutritional Information (per serving, approximate):

Calories: 400 kcal| Protein: 15 g| Fat: 15 g (Saturated: 5 g, Unsaturated: 10 g)| Carbohydrates: 55 g (Fiber: 10 g, Sugars: 8 g)| Cholesterol: 185 mg| Sodium: 600 mg

LUNCH RECIPES:

RECIPES 1

TURMERIC CAULIFLOWER SOUP WITH A SIDE OF WHOLE GRAIN BREAD

Serves: 4 servings | Prep Time: 10 minutes | Cooking Time: 20 minutes | Total Time: 30 minutes

Ingredients:

For the Soup:

- 1 large head of cauliflower, cut into florets

- 1 tablespoon olive oil

- 1 medium onion, diced

- 2 cloves garlic, minced

- 1 teaspoon ground turmeric

- 4 cups vegetable broth

- Salt and pepper, to taste

- 1 cup coconut milk (for creaminess, optional)

- Fresh cilantro or parsley, for garnish

For Serving:

- 4 slices of whole grain bread

Instructions:

1. Sauté the Vegetables: Heat olive oil in a large pot over medium heat. Add the diced onion and minced garlic, sautéing until the onion is translucent and fragrant, about 3-5 minutes. Add the ground turmeric and stir for another minute until the spices are fragrant.

2. Cook the Cauliflower: Add the cauliflower florets to the pot and stir until they are well-coated with the turmeric and onion mixture. After adding the veggie broth, heat the mixture until it boils. Let it simmer for about 15-20

minutes, or until the cauliflower is tender.

3. Blend the Soup: Once the cauliflower is soft, use an immersion blender to blend the soup directly in the pot until smooth. Alternatively, you can transfer the soup in batches to a blender and blend until smooth, then return it to the pot. If using coconut milk for creaminess, stir it into the soup after blending.

4. Season and Serve: Taste the soup and adjust the seasoning with salt and pepper as needed. After the pot reaches a boil, lower the heat to a simmer and cover it. Serve each bowl of soup with a slice of whole grain bread on the side.

Nutritional Information (per serving, approximate):

Calories: 250 kcal| Protein: 6 g| Fat: 14 g (Saturated: 7 g, Unsaturated: 7 g)| Carbohydrates: 28 g (Fiber: 6 g, Sugars: 8 g) |

Cholesterol: 0 mg| Sodium: 800 mg

RECIPE 2

ZUCCHINI NOODLES WITH PESTO AND CHERRY TOMATOES

Serves: 2 servings| Prep Time: 15 minutes| Cooking Time: 0 minutes (no cooking required for the noodles) | Total Time: 15 minutes

Ingredients:

- 2 medium zucchinis

- 1 cup cherry tomatoes, halved

- 1/4 cup pesto (homemade or store-bought)

- Salt and pepper, to taste

- Optional: Grated Parmesan cheese for garnish

- Optional: Fresh basil leaves for garnish

Instructions:

1. Prepare Zucchini Noodles: Wash the zucchinis and cut the ends off. Use a spiralizer to turn the zucchinis into noodles. If you don't have a spiralizer, you can use a julienne peeler or a regular peeler to make wide ribbons.

2. Mix with Pesto: In a large bowl, combine the zucchini noodles and pesto. Toss gently until the noodles are well-coated with the pesto. Season with salt and pepper to taste.

3. Add Cherry Tomatoes: Gently fold in the halved cherry tomatoes, being careful not to break them.

4. Serve: Divide the zucchini noodles between two plates. If desired, garnish with grated Parmesan cheese and fresh basil leaves.

5. Enjoy: Serve immediately as a fresh and light meal. For a heartier dish, you might add grilled chicken or shrimp on top.

Nutritional Information (per serving, approximate):

Calories: 180 kcal| Protein: 5 g| Fat: 14 g (Saturated: 3 g, Unsaturated: 11 g)| Carbohydrates: 10 g (Fiber: 3 g, Sugars: 6 g)| Cholesterol: 5 mg| Sodium: 250 mg

RECIPE 3

Stuffed Bell Peppers with Quinoa, Black Beans, and Corn

Serves: 4 servings| Prep Time: 20 minutes| Cooking Time: 45 minutes| Total Time: 1 hour and 5 minutes

Ingredients:

- 4 large bell peppers (any color)

- 1 cup quinoa, rinsed and drained

- 2 cups vegetable broth (for cooking quinoa)

- 1 can (15 oz) black beans, drained and rinsed

- 1 cup corn kernels (fresh, frozen, or canned)

- 1 cup diced tomatoes (canned or fresh)

- 1/2 cup diced red onion

- 2 cloves garlic, minced

- 1 teaspoon ground cumin

- 1 teaspoon chili powder

- Salt and pepper, to taste

- 1 cup shredded cheese (cheddar, Monterey Jack, or your choice)

- Fresh cilantro or parsley, for garnish (optional)

Instructions:

1. Prepare the Quinoa: In a medium saucepan, combine the quinoa and vegetable broth. Bring to a boil, then reduce the heat to low, cover, and simmer for 15-20 minutes, or until the quinoa is cooked and the liquid is absorbed. Fluff with a fork and set aside.

2. Prepare the Bell Peppers: Cut the tops off

the bell peppers and remove the seeds and membranes from the inside. If needed, trim the bottoms slightly to ensure they stand upright in a baking dish. Place the hollowed-out bell peppers in a baking dish and set aside.

3. Prepare the Filling: In a large skillet, heat a bit of olive oil over medium heat. Add the diced red onion and minced garlic, sautéing for about 2-3 minutes until they soften. Add the diced tomatoes, black beans, corn, ground cumin, chili powder, salt, and pepper. Cook for an additional 2-3 minutes to combine the flavors. Remove the skillet from heat, and fold in the cooked quinoa. Mix until everything is well combined.

4. Stuff the Bell Peppers: Set your oven to 350°F (175°C). Carefully stuff each bell pepper with the quinoa and vegetable mixture. Press down gently to pack the filling.

5. Bake: Place the stuffed bell peppers in the preheated oven and bake for 30-35 minutes, or until the peppers are tender.

6. Add Cheese and Finish: Remove the baking dish from the oven. Sprinkle shredded cheese over the tops of the stuffed peppers. Return the dish to the oven and bake for an additional 10 minutes, or until the cheese is melted and bubbly.

7. Serve: Garnish with fresh cilantro or parsley if desired. Serve the Stuffed Bell Peppers hot, and enjoy!

Nutritional Information (per serving, approximate):

Calories: 400 kcal| Protein: 16 g| Fat: 11 g (Saturated: 5 g, Unsaturated: 6 g)| Carbohydrates: 65 g (Fiber: 14 g, Sugars: 6 g) | Cholesterol: 20 mg| Sodium: 600 mg

BEETROOT AND GOAT CHEESE ARUGULA SALAD

Serves: 4 servings

Prep Time: 15 minutes (plus time to roast beets if using fresh)

Cooking Time: 60 minutes for roasting beets (if using fresh)

Total Time: 1 hour 15 minutes (with pre-roasted or canned beets, it's just 15 minutes)

Ingredients:

- 4 medium beetroots (or you can use pre-cooked beets for convenience)

- 4 cups arugula, washed and dried

- 1/2 cup goat cheese, crumbled

- 1/4 cup walnuts, toasted and chopped

- 2 tablespoons balsamic vinegar

- 4 tablespoons olive oil

- Salt and pepper, to taste

- Optional: 1 teaspoon honey or maple syrup to sweeten the dressing

Instructions:

1. Roast the Beets (if using fresh):

   - Pre-Set your oven to 400°F (200°C).

   - Wash and trim the beetroots, wrap them individually in foil, and place them on a baking sheet.

   - Roast in the preheated oven for about 1 hour

or until tender when pierced with a fork. Allow them to cool, then peel and slice into wedges or cubes.

2. Prepare the Dressing:

- In a small bowl, whisk together balsamic vinegar, olive oil, salt, pepper, and optional honey or maple syrup for a slightly sweetened dressing.

3. Assemble the Salad:

- In a large bowl, gently toss the arugula with half of the dressing.

- Carefully place the dressed arugula on individual plates or serving platter.

- Top with roasted beet wedges or cubes, crumbled goat cheese, and toasted walnuts.

4. Dress the Salad: Drizzle the remaining dressing over the salad just before serving.

5. Serve: Enjoy this vibrant salad as a fresh starter or a light meal.

Nutritional Information (per serving, approximate):

Calories: 250 kcal| Protein: 7 g| Fat: 20 g (Saturated: 5 g, Unsaturated: 15 g)| Carbohydrates: 12 g (Fiber: 3 g, Sugars: 8 g)| Cholesterol: 13 mg| Sodium: 200 mg

RECIPE 5

ASIAN-STYLE TOFU STIR-FRY WITH BROWN RICE AND MIXED VEGETABLES

Serves: 4 servings| Prep Time: 15 minutes|

Cooking Time: 20 minutes| Total Time: 35 minutes

Ingredients:

For the Stir-fry:

- 14 oz (400g) firm tofu, cubed

- 2 cups mixed vegetables (e.g., bell peppers, broccoli, carrots, snap peas), chopped

- 2 cloves garlic, minced

- 1 tablespoon fresh ginger, minced

- 2 tablespoons vegetable oil (for stir-frying)

- Salt and pepper, to taste

- Optional: Red pepper flakes for heat

For the Sauce:

- 1/4 cup low-sodium soy sauce

- 2 tablespoons hoisin sauce

- 1 tablespoon rice vinegar

- 1 tablespoon honey or maple syrup

- 1 teaspoon cornstarch (to thicken the sauce)

For Serving:

- 2 cups cooked brown rice (prepared according to package instructions)

- Optional garnish: sliced green onions, sesame seeds

Instructions:

1. Prepare the Sauce: In a small bowl, whisk together the soy sauce, hoisin sauce, rice vinegar, honey or maple syrup, and cornstarch. Set the sauce aside.

2. Prepare the Tofu: If using extra-firm tofu,

press it to remove excess moisture. You can do this by wrapping the tofu block in a clean kitchen towel and placing something heavy on top, like a skillet. Leave it for about 10-15 minutes, then cube the tofu. Heat 1 tablespoon of vegetable oil in a large skillet or wok over medium-high heat. Add the tofu cubes and cook until they are golden brown on all sides. Remove the tofu from the skillet and set it aside.

3. Stir-fry Vegetables: In the same skillet, add the remaining tablespoon of vegetable oil. Add minced garlic and ginger, and stir-fry for about 30 seconds until fragrant. Add the chopped mixed vegetables and stir-fry for about 5-7 minutes, or until they are tender-crisp.

4. Combine Tofu and Sauce: Return the cooked tofu to the skillet with the vegetables. Pour the prepared sauce over the tofu and vegetables. Stir well to coat everything evenly. Cook for an

additional 2-3 minutes, or until the sauce thickens.

5. Serve: Divide the cooked brown rice among four plates.

   - Spoon the tofu and vegetable stir-fry over the rice.

   - Garnish with sliced green onions and sesame seeds if desired.

6. Enjoy: Serve your Asian-style Tofu Stir-fry hot, and enjoy this flavorful and wholesome meal!

Nutritional Information (per serving, approximate):

Calories: 350 kcal| Protein: 14 g| Fat: 14 g (Saturated: 1 g, Unsaturated: 13 g)| Carbohydrates: 45 g (Fiber: 6 g, Sugars: 10 g)| Cholesterol: 0 mg| Sodium: 700 mg

GRILLED CHICKEN AND QUINOA SALAD WITH AVOCADO AND CUCUMBER

Serves: 4 servings | Prep Time: 15 minutes | Cooking Time: 20 minutes (for quinoa and chicken) | Total Time: 35 minutes

Ingredients:

For the Salad:

- 2 boneless, skinless chicken breasts

- 1 cup quinoa

- 2 cups water or chicken broth (for cooking quinoa)

- 2 ripe avocados, diced

- 1 cucumber, diced

- 1 cup cherry tomatoes, halved

- 1/2 red onion, finely chopped

- 1/4 cup fresh cilantro or parsley, chopped

For the Dressing:

- 3 tablespoons olive oil

- 2 tablespoons lemon juice

- 1 clove garlic, minced

- Salt and pepper, to taste

Instructions:

1. Cook the Quinoa: Rinse the quinoa under cold water and drain. In a saucepan, combine the quinoa and water or chicken broth. Bring to a

boil. Reduce the heat to low, cover, and simmer for 15-20 minutes, or until the quinoa is cooked and the liquid is absorbed. Fluff with a fork and let it cool.

2. Grill the Chicken: Preheat your grill or grill pan over medium-high heat. Season the chicken breasts with salt and pepper. Grill the chicken for about 6-8 minutes per side, or until cooked through and no longer pink in the center. Remove from the grill, let it rest for a few minutes, then slice it into thin strips.

3. Prepare the Dressing: In a small bowl, whisk together the olive oil, lemon juice, minced garlic, salt, and pepper. Set aside.

4. Assemble the Salad: In a large salad bowl, combine the cooked and cooled quinoa, diced avocados, diced cucumber, halved cherry tomatoes, finely chopped red onion, and chopped cilantro or parsley. Add the sliced

grilled chicken on top.

5. Dress the Salad: Drizzle the dressing over the salad and gently toss everything together until well combined.

6. Serve: Divide the Grilled Chicken and Quinoa Salad into four servings and serve it as a healthy and satisfying meal.

Nutritional Information (per serving, approximate):

Calories: 450 kcal| Protein: 30 g| Fat: 25 g (Saturated: 4 g, Unsaturated: 21 g)| Carbohydrates: 30 g (Fiber: 9 g, Sugars: 4 g)| Cholesterol: 70 mg| Sodium: 250 mg

RECIPE 7

ROASTED VEGETABLE AND CHICKPEA WRAP WITH HUMMUS

Serves: 4 servings | Prep Time: 15 minutes | Cooking Time: 25 minutes (for roasting vegetables) | Total Time: 40 minutes

Ingredients:

For the Roasted Vegetables:

- 2 cups mixed vegetables (e.g., bell peppers, zucchini, cherry tomatoes), chopped

- 1 can (15 oz) chickpeas, drained and rinsed

- 2 tablespoons olive oil

- 1 teaspoon dried oregano

- Salt and pepper, to taste

For the Wraps:

- 4 whole wheat or spinach tortillas

- 1 cup hummus (store-bought or homemade)

- 1 cup baby spinach leaves

- 1/2 cup feta cheese, crumbled (optional)

- Optional additional toppings: sliced olives, cucumber, red onion, or avocado

Instructions:

1. Preheat the Oven: Set your oven to 425°F (220°C).

2. Roast the Vegetables and Chickpeas: In a large mixing bowl, combine the chopped mixed vegetables, chickpeas, olive oil, dried oregano, salt, and pepper. Toss everything together to coat evenly. On your baking sheet, spread the

mixture in a single layer. In the preheated oven, roast the vegetables for 20-25 minutes time, or until they become tender and slightly caramelized. Stir occasionally for even cooking.

3. Assemble the Wraps: While the vegetables are roasting, warm the tortillas in a dry skillet or microwave for a few seconds to make them more pliable. Spread a generous layer of hummus on each tortilla.

4. Add Roasted Vegetables and Chickpeas: Once the vegetables and chickpeas are roasted to perfection, remove them from the oven. Divide the roasted mixture evenly among the tortillas, placing it on top of the hummus.

5. Add Spinach and Optional Toppings: Top each wrap with a handful of baby spinach leaves and crumbled feta cheese (if using). If desired, add additional toppings such as sliced olives, cucumber, red onion, or avocado.

6. Fold and Serve: Fold the sides of each tortilla in and then roll it up tightly to form a wrap.

7. Enjoy: Serve the Roasted Vegetable and Chickpea Wraps immediately, and enjoy this flavorful and nutritious meal!

Nutritional Information (per serving, approximate):

Calories: 400 kcal| Protein: 15 g| Fat: 18 g (Saturated: 3 g, Unsaturated: 15 g)| Carbohydrates: 45 g (Fiber: 10 g, Sugars: 3 g| Cholesterol: 0 mg| Sodium: 700 mg

RECIPE 8

LENTIL AND SPINACH STEW WITH

BROWN RICE

Serves: 4 servings| Prep Time: 10 minutes| Cooking Time: 30 minutes| Total Time: 40 minutes

Ingredients:

- 1 cup brown lentils, rinsed and drained

- 1 cup brown rice

- 4 cups vegetable broth

- 1 onion, chopped

- 2 cloves garlic, minced

- 2 carrots, peeled and diced

- 2 celery stalks, diced

- 1 can (15 oz) diced tomatoes

- 2 cups fresh spinach, chopped

- 1 teaspoon ground cumin

- 1 teaspoon ground coriander

- Salt and pepper, to taste

- 2 tablespoons olive oil

- Optional garnish: Fresh cilantro or parsley

Instructions:

1. Cook the Brown Rice: In a separate saucepan, cook the brown rice according to the package instructions. This usually involves combining 1 cup of rice with 2 cups of water or vegetable broth, bringing it to a boil, then reducing the heat, covering, and simmering for about 45 minutes or until the rice is tender. Set it aside when done.

2. Sauté the Vegetables: In a large pot, heat the olive oil over medium heat. Add the chopped onion, minced garlic, diced carrots, and diced

celery. Sauté for about 5 minutes until the vegetables start to soften.

3. Add Lentils and Spices: Add the rinsed and drained brown lentils, ground cumin, ground coriander, salt, and pepper to the pot with the sautéed vegetables. Stir to combine.

4. Add Broth and Tomatoes: Pour in the vegetable broth and diced tomatoes. Stir everything together.

5. Simmer the Stew: Bring the mixture to a boil, then reduce the heat to a simmer. Cover the pot and let it simmer for about 20-25 minutes, or until the lentils are tender.

6. Add Spinach: Stir in the chopped fresh spinach and cook for an additional 2-3 minutes until the spinach wilts.

7. Serve: To serve, place a scoop of cooked brown rice in each bowl, then ladle the lentil and

spinach stew over the rice.

8. Garnish: If desired, garnish with fresh cilantro or parsley.

9. Enjoy: Serve the Lentil and Spinach Stew with Brown Rice hot and enjoy this wholesome and comforting meal!

Nutritional Information (per serving, approximate):

Calories: 350 kcal| Protein: 13 g| Fat: 6 g (Saturated: 1 g, Unsaturated: 5 g)| Carbohydrates: 61 g (Fiber: 11 g, Sugars: 6 g)| Cholesterol: 0 mg| Sodium: 700 mg

RECIPE 9

Baked Salmon with Steamed Broccoli and Sweet Potato Mash:

Serves: 4 servings | Prep Time: 15 minutes | Cooking Time: 25 minutes | Total Time: 40 minutes

Ingredients:

For the Baked Salmon:

- 4 salmon fillets (about 6 oz each)

- 2 tablespoons olive oil

- 2 cloves garlic, minced

- 1 lemon, thinly sliced

- Salt and pepper, to taste

- Fresh dill or parsley, for garnish (optional)

For the Steamed Broccoli:

- 4 cups broccoli florets

For the Sweet Potato Mash:

- 2 large sweet potatoes, peeled and cubed

- 2 tablespoons butter or olive oil

- Salt and pepper, to taste

- Optional: a pinch of nutmeg or cinnamon for extra flavor

Instructions:

1. Preheat the Oven: Pre-Set your oven to 375°F (190°C).

2. Prepare the Salmon: - Place the salmon fillets on a baking sheet lined with parchment paper. Drizzle olive oil over the salmon, then sprinkle minced garlic, salt, and pepper evenly over each fillet. Top each fillet with lemon slices for added flavor.

3. Bake the Salmon: Bake the salmon in the preheated oven for about 15-20 minutes, or until the salmon flakes easily with a fork and is cooked to your desired level of doneness.

4. Steam the Broccoli: While the salmon is baking, steam the broccoli florets until they are tender but still crisp, about 5-7 minutes. You can use a steamer basket or microwave for this.

5. Prepare the Sweet Potato Mash:

  - In a separate pot, boil the sweet potato cubes until they are tender, about 10-15 minutes.

  - Drain the sweet potatoes and return them to the pot.

  - Mash the sweet potatoes with butter or olive oil, salt, pepper, and optionally a pinch of nutmeg or cinnamon for extra flavor.

6. Serve: Plate each serving with a baked

salmon fillet, steamed broccoli, and a scoop of sweet potato mash.

7. Garnish: If desired, garnish the salmon with fresh dill or parsley for a pop of color and flavor.

8. Enjoy; Serve your Baked Salmon with Steamed Broccoli and Sweet Potato Mash hot, and savor this nutritious and satisfying meal!

Nutritional Information (per serving, approximate):

Calories: 400 kcal| Protein: 30 g| Fat: 18 g (Saturated: 5 g, Unsaturated: 13 g) | Carbohydrates: 30 g (Fiber: 6 g, Sugars: 7 g) | Cholesterol: 70 mg| Sodium: 200 mg

Note: Nutritional values are approximate and can vary based on the specific brands and types of ingredients used, as well as any modifications to the recipe. This Baked Salmon with Steamed Broccoli and Sweet Potato Mash is a well-balanced meal with lean protein, healthy fats, and nutrient-rich vegetables. It's both delicious and nutritious.

RECIPE 10

Kale, Strawberry, and Walnut Salad with Grilled Tofu

Serves: 4 servings | Prep Time: 20 minutes | Cooking Time: 10 minutes (for grilling tofu) | Total Time: 30 minutes

Ingredients:

For the Salad:

- 8 cups kale leaves, washed and chopped

- 2 cups fresh strawberries, hulled and sliced

- 1/2 cup walnuts, chopped

- 1/4 cup red onion, thinly sliced

- 1/4 cup crumbled feta cheese (optional)

- 1/4 cup dried cranberries (optional)

For the Grilled Tofu:

- 1 block (14 oz) extra-firm tofu, pressed and sliced into 1/2-inch thick pieces

- 2 tablespoons olive oil

- 1 lemon, juiced

- 1 teaspoon dried oregano

- Salt and pepper, to taste

For the Dressing:

- 3 tablespoons olive oil

- 2 tablespoons balsamic vinegar

- 1 tablespoon honey or maple syrup (for sweetness)

- Salt and pepper, to taste

Instructions:

1. Prepare the Tofu: press the tofu to remove excess moisture. You can do this by wrapping the tofu block in a clean kitchen towel and placing something heavy on top, like a skillet. Leave it for about 10-15 minutes. Slice the pressed tofu into 1/2-inch thick pieces. In a bowl, whisk together 2 tablespoons of olive oil, lemon juice, dried oregano, salt, and pepper. Marinate the tofu slices in this mixture for about 10 minutes.

2. Grill the Tofu: Preheat your grill or grill pan over medium-high heat. Grill the marinated tofu slices for about 3-5 minutes on each side, or until they have grill marks and are heated through. Set aside.

3. Prepare the Salad: In a large salad bowl, combine the chopped kale, sliced strawberries, chopped walnuts, thinly sliced red onion, crumbled feta cheese (if using), and dried cranberries (if using).

4. Prepare the Dressing: In a small bowl, whisk together 3 tablespoons of olive oil, balsamic vinegar, honey or maple syrup for sweetness, salt, and pepper.

5. Assemble the Salad: Drizzle the dressing over the salad ingredients. Toss everything together to coat the salad evenly with the dressing.

6. Add Grilled Tofu: Place the grilled tofu slices on top of the salad.

7. Serve: Serve the Kale, Strawberry, and Walnut Salad with Grilled Tofu immediately, and enjoy this healthy and flavorful meal!

Nutritional Information (per serving, approximate):

Calories: 400 kcal| Protein: 14 g| Fat: 27 g (Saturated: 4 g, Unsaturated: 23 g)| Carbohydrates: 33 g (Fiber: 5 g, Sugars: 14 g)| Cholesterol: 5 mg| Sodium: 300 mg

DINNER RECIPES

RECIPE 1

BAKED COD WITH A LEMON HERB CRUST AND ROASTED ASPARAGUS

This recipe offers a delightful combination of tender, flaky cod with a zesty lemon herb crust, paired with perfectly roasted asparagus. It's a nutritious and delicious meal that's easy to prepare, making it perfect for a weeknight dinner or a special occasion.

Serves: 4 servings | Prep Time: 15 minutes | Cooking Time: 20 minutes | Total Time: 35 minutes

Ingredients:

For the Cod:

- 4 cod fillets (about 6 ounces each)

- 2 tablespoons olive oil

- 1 tablespoon lemon zest

- 2 tablespoons fresh lemon juice

- 2 garlic cloves, minced

- 1/2 cup panko breadcrumbs

- 2 tablespoons fresh parsley, chopped

- 1 tablespoon fresh thyme, chopped

- Salt and pepper, to taste

For the Asparagus:

- 1 pound asparagus, ends trimmed

- 1 tablespoon olive oil

- Salt and pepper, to taste

- Lemon wedges, for serving

Instructions:

1. Preheat Oven and Prepare Baking Sheet: Set your oven to 400°F (200°C). Line a baking sheet with parchment paper or lightly grease it.

2. Season the Cod: In a small bowl, mix 1 tablespoon of olive oil, lemon zest, and lemon juice. Place the cod fillets on the prepared baking sheet and brush them with the lemon olive oil mixture. Season with salt and pepper.

3. Prepare the Lemon Herb Crust: In another bowl, combine the panko breadcrumbs, parsley, thyme, minced garlic, and the remaining tablespoon of olive oil. Mix until the breadcrumbs are well moistened. Press this mixture onto the top of each cod fillet, forming a crust.

4. Prepare Asparagus: On another baking sheet,

toss the asparagus with 1 tablespoon of olive oil, salt, and pepper. Spread them out in a single layer.

5. Bake Cod and Asparagus: Place both the cod and asparagus in the oven. Bake for about 12-15 minutes, or until the cod is flaky and cooked through, and the asparagus is tender and slightly crisp.

6. Serve: Remove from the oven. Serve the baked cod and roasted asparagus hot, with lemon wedges on the side for added zest.

Nutritional Information (per serving):

Calories: 280| Protein: 30g| Carbohydrates: 12g| Fat: 12g| Saturated Fat: 2g| Cholesterol: 60mg| Sodium: 200mg| Fiber: 2g| Sugar: 2g

RECIPE 2

MOROCCAN LENTIL AND SWEET POTATO STEW

This hearty and aromatic stew combines the earthy flavors of lentils with the natural sweetness of sweet potatoes, infused with a vibrant mix of Moroccan spices. It's a comforting and nutritious dish, perfect for chilly evenings or whenever you're in the mood for something flavorful and satisfying.

Serves: 6 servings| Prep Time: 15 minutes| Cooking Time: 40 minutes| Total Time: 55 minutes

Ingredients:

- 1 tablespoon olive oil

- 1 large onion, diced

- 3 garlic cloves, minced

- 2 teaspoons ground cumin

- 1 teaspoon ground coriander

- 1/2 teaspoon ground cinnamon

- 1/4 teaspoon ground turmeric

- 1/4 teaspoon cayenne pepper (adjust to taste)

- 2 sweet potatoes (about 1 pound), peeled and cut into 1/2-inch cubes

- 1 cup dried lentils (green or brown), rinsed and drained

- 4 cups vegetable broth

- 1 can (14 ounces) diced tomatoes, with their juice

- 1 teaspoon salt (adjust to taste)

- 1/2 teaspoon freshly ground black pepper

- 3 cups baby spinach leaves

- 1/4 cup chopped fresh cilantro, plus more for garnish

- Juice of 1 lemon

Instructions:

1. Sauté Aromatics: Heat the olive oil in a large pot over medium heat. Add the onion and garlic, sautéing until the onion is translucent and fragrant, about 5 minutes.

2. Add Spices: Stir in the cumin, coriander, cinnamon, turmeric, and cayenne pepper. Cook for another minute until the spices are fragrant.

3. Combine Ingredients: Add the sweet potatoes,

lentils, vegetable broth, and diced tomatoes (with their juice) to the pot. Season with salt and pepper. Stir well to combine all the ingredients.

4. Simmer the Stew: Bring the mixture to a boil, then reduce the heat to low. Cover and simmer for about 30 minutes, or until the lentils and sweet potatoes are tender.

5. Add Spinach and Final Touches**: Stir in the spinach and cook until it's wilted, about 2 minutes. Remove the pot from the heat and stir in the chopped cilantro and lemon juice.

6. Serve: Taste and adjust seasoning if necessary. Serve the stew hot, garnished with additional cilantro if desired.

Nutritional Information (per serving):

Calories: 220| Protein: 11g| Carbohydrates:

40g| Fat: 3g| Saturated Fat: 0.5g|Sodium: 750mg| Fiber: 15g|Sugar: 8g

RECIPE 3

STUFFED ACORN SQUASH WITH WILD RICE AND CRANBERRIES

This dish features roasted acorn squash filled with a savory blend of wild rice, cranberries, nuts, and herbs, creating a delightful mix of textures and flavors. It's a visually stunning dish that works well as a hearty main course or an elegant side.

Serves: 4 servings| Prep Time: 20 minutes| Cooking Time: 60 minutes| Total Time: 1 hour 20 minutes

Ingredients:

For the Squash:

- 2 acorn squashes, halved and seeds removed

- 2 tablespoons olive oil

- Salt and pepper, to taste

For the Filling:

- 1 cup wild rice blend, rinsed

- 2 1/4 cups vegetable broth or water

- 1/2 cup dried cranberries

- 1/2 cup pecans or walnuts, chopped (optional)

- 1 medium onion, diced

- 2 cloves garlic, minced

- 2 celery stalks, diced

- 1 carrot, diced

- 1 teaspoon dried thyme

- 1/2 teaspoon dried sage

- Salt and pepper, to taste

- 2 tablespoons fresh parsley, chopped (for garnish)

Instructions:

1. Roast the Squash: Set your oven to 375°F (190°C). Brush the cut sides of the acorn squash with olive oil and season with salt and pepper. Place them cut-side down on a baking sheet and roast until tender, about 40-45 minutes.

2. Cook the Wild Rice: While the squash is roasting, combine the wild rice blend and vegetable broth in a medium saucepan. Bring to a boil, then reduce the heat to low, cover, and

simmer until the rice is tender and the liquid is absorbed, about 45 minutes.

3. Prepare the Filling: In a large skillet, heat a tablespoon of olive oil over medium heat. Add the onion, garlic, celery, and carrot, sautéing until softened, about 5-7 minutes. Stir in the dried thyme and sage, and cook for an additional minute.

4. Combine Ingredients: Mix the cooked wild rice, sautéed vegetables, dried cranberries, and nuts (if using) in a large bowl. Season with salt and pepper to taste.

5. Stuff the Squash: Once the squash halves are roasted and tender, fill them with the wild rice mixture. Return them to the oven for about 10 minutes, or until everything is heated through.

6. Serve: Garnish the stuffed squashes with chopped parsley before serving.

Nutritional Information (per serving):

Calories: 350| Protein: 8g| Carbohydrates: 60g| Fat: 12g| Saturated Fat: 1.5g| Sodium: 300mg| Fiber: 8g| Sugar: 15g

RECIPE 4

GRILLED EGGPLANT AND BELL PEPPER STACK WITH BASIL PESTO

This vibrant and flavorful dish layers grilled eggplant and bell peppers with a homemade basil pesto, creating a stunning presentation. It's a light yet satisfying meal that highlights the fresh tastes of summer.

Serves: 4 servings | Prep Time: 20 minutes (plus time for pesto if making from scratch)

Cooking Time: 15 minutes

Total Time: 35 minutes (plus additional for pesto)

Ingredients:

For the Vegetables:

- 2 large eggplants, sliced into 1/2-inch rounds

- 2 red bell peppers, quartered

- 2 yellow bell peppers, quartered

- 2 tablespoons olive oil

- Salt and pepper, to taste

For the Basil Pesto:

- 2 cups fresh basil leaves

- 1/2 cup grated Parmesan cheese

- 1/3 cup pine nuts or walnuts

- 2 garlic cloves

- 1/2 cup extra-virgin olive oil

- Salt and pepper, to taste

Instructions:

1. Prep the Vegetables: Preheat your grill or grill pan to medium-high heat. Brush both sides of the eggplant slices and bell pepper quarters with olive oil, and season with salt and pepper.

2. Grill the Vegetables: Grill the eggplant slices for about 4-5 minutes per side, or until tender and grill marks appear. Grill the bell peppers, skin-side down, for about 5-6 minutes, or until the skin is charred and they're tender. Remove the vegetables from the grill and set aside. Once

cool enough to handle, peel the skins off the bell peppers.

3. Make the Basil Pesto: In a food processor, combine the basil leaves, Parmesan cheese, nuts, and garlic. Pulse until coarsely chopped. While the processor is running, slowly add the olive oil and process until fully integrated and smooth. Season with salt and pepper to taste.

4. Assemble the Stacks: On a serving plate, start with a slice of grilled eggplant, add a layer of grilled bell pepper, and then a generous spread of basil pesto. Repeat the layers until you've formed a stack. Repeat this process to make four individual stacks.

5. Serve: Serve the stacks immediately, garnished with additional basil leaves or a drizzle of olive oil if desired.

Nutritional Information (per serving):

Calories: 380| Protein: 8g| Carbohydrates: 20g| Fat: 32g| Saturated Fat: 5g| Cholesterol: 10mg| Sodium: 250mg| Fiber: 8g| Sugar: 12g

RECIPE 5

GINGER SOY GLAZED SALMON WITH STEAMED BOK CHOY AND BROWN RICE

This dish combines the rich flavors of ginger and soy sauce glazed salmon with the subtle, earthy tones of steamed bok choy and nutty brown rice. It's a well-balanced meal that's both nutritious and satisfying, perfect for a wholesome dinner.

Serves: 4 servings| Prep Time: 15 minutes| Cooking Time:| 30 minutes| Total Time: 45 minutes

Ingredients:

For the Salmon:

- 4 salmon fillets (about 6 ounces each)

- 2 tablespoons soy sauce

- 1 tablespoon fresh ginger, minced

- 2 garlic cloves, minced

- 2 tablespoons honey

- 1 tablespoon olive oil

- 1 teaspoon sesame oil

For the Bok Choy:

- 4 heads of bok choy, halved or quartered

- 1 tablespoon olive oil

- Salt and pepper, to taste

For the Brown Rice:

- 1 cup brown rice

- 2 1/4 cups water

- Salt, to taste

Instructions:

1. Cook the Brown Rice: Rinse the brown rice under cold water. In a medium saucepan, bring the water to a boil. Add the rinsed rice and a pinch of salt, then reduce the heat to low. Cover and simmer for about 45 minutes, or until the water is absorbed and the rice is tender. Remove from heat and let it sit, covered, for 5 minutes.

2. Prep the Salmon Glaze: In a small bowl, whisk together the soy sauce, minced ginger, minced garlic, honey, olive oil, and sesame oil.

3. Marinate the Salmon: Place the salmon fillets in a shallow dish and pour the ginger soy glaze over them, ensuring they are well coated. Let them marinate for at least 10 minutes.

4. Cook the Salmon: Preheat your grill, grill pan, or broiler. Grill or broil the salmon fillets for about 4-5 minutes per side, or until they are just cooked through and easily flake with a fork. During the last few minutes of cooking, brush the fillets with any remaining glaze to enhance the flavor.

5. Steam the Bok Choy: While the salmon is cooking, heat 1 tablespoon of olive oil in a large skillet over medium heat. Add the bok choy, cut-side down, and cook for 2-3 minutes until it starts to sear. Add a splash of water to the pan

and cover it, allowing the bok choy to steam for about 3-4 minutes, or until tender. Season with salt and pepper to taste.

6. Serve: Spoon a serving of brown rice onto each plate, top with a salmon fillet, and arrange the steamed bok choy on the side.

Nutritional Information (per serving):

Calories: 500| Protein: 36g| Carbohydrates: 45g| Fat: 20g| Saturated Fat: 3g| Cholesterol: 75mg| Sodium: 600mg| Fiber: 4g| Sugar: 10g

RECIPE 6

SPINACH AND FETA STUFFED CHICKEN

BREAST WITH QUINOA SALAD

This dish combines juicy, spinach and feta stuffed chicken breasts with a light and refreshing quinoa salad. It's a healthy and flavorful meal that's perfect for any day of the week.

Serves: 4 servings| Prep Time: 20 minutes| Cooking Time: 30 minutes| Total Time: 50 minutes

Ingredients:

For the Stuffed Chicken:

- 4 boneless, skinless chicken breasts

- 1 cup fresh spinach, chopped

- 1/2 cup feta cheese, crumbled

- 2 cloves garlic, minced

- 1 tablespoon olive oil

- Salt and pepper, to taste

- Toothpicks or kitchen twine (for securing chicken)

For the Quinoa Salad:

- 1 cup quinoa

- 2 cups water

- 1 cup cherry tomatoes, halved

- 1 cucumber, diced

- 1/4 cup red onion, finely chopped

- 1/4 cup fresh parsley, chopped

- 2 tablespoons lemon juice

- 2 tablespoons olive oil

- Salt and pepper, to taste

Instructions:

1. Prepare the Quinoa Salad: Rinse the quinoa under cold water. In a medium saucepan, bring 2 cups of water to a boil. Add the quinoa and a pinch of salt, reduce the heat to low, cover, and simmer for about 15 minutes, or until the water is absorbed. Remove from heat and let it sit, covered, for 5 minutes. Fluff with a fork and let it cool. Once cooled, add the cherry tomatoes, cucumber, red onion, parsley, lemon juice, and olive oil. Toss to combine and season with salt and pepper to taste.

2. Preheat the Oven: Set your oven to 375°F (190°C).

3. Prepare the Chicken: Make a horizontal cut along the side of each chicken breast to create a

pocket, being careful not to cut all the way through. In a bowl, mix the chopped spinach, crumbled feta, minced garlic, salt, and pepper. Stuff each chicken breast with the spinach and feta mixture, then secure the openings with toothpicks or kitchen twine.

4. Cook the Chicken: Heat 1 tablespoon of olive oil in an ovenproof skillet over medium-high heat. Sear the chicken breasts on each side until golden brown, about 3-4 minutes per side. Transfer the skillet to the oven and bake for 20 -25 minutes, or until the chicken is cooked through and the juices run clear.

5. Serve: Remove the toothpicks or twine from the chicken, slice if desired, and serve alongside the quinoa salad.

Nutritional Information (per serving):

Calories: 450| Protein: 38g| Carbohydrates: 40g| Fat: 16g| Saturated Fat: 4g| Cholesterol: 100mg| Sodium: 400mg| Fiber: 5g| Sugar: 3g

RECIPE 7

BUTTERNUT SQUASH AND CHICKPEA CURRY WITH BROWN BASMATI RICE

This warming and hearty curry combines the sweetness of butternut squash with the richness of chickpeas, all simmered in a fragrant blend of spices and served over nutty brown basmati rice. It's a comforting and nutritious meal that's perfect for a cozy night in.

Serves:4 servings| Prep Time: 15 minutes| Cooking Time: 45 minutes| Total Time: 1 hour

Ingredients:

For the Curry:

- 1 tablespoon coconut oil

- 1 large onion, diced

- 3 garlic cloves, minced

- 1 tablespoon fresh ginger, minced

- 1 tablespoon garam masala

- 1 teaspoon ground turmeric

- 1 teaspoon ground cumin

- 1/2 teaspoon chili powder (adjust to taste)

- 1 medium butternut squash, peeled and cut into 1-inch cubes

- 1 can (15 ounces) chickpeas, drained and rinsed

- 1 can (14 ounces) coconut milk

- 1 cup vegetable broth

- Salt and pepper, to taste

- Fresh cilantro, chopped (for garnish)

For the Brown Basmati Rice:

- 1 cup brown basmati rice

- 2 1/2 cups water

- Salt, to taste

Instructions:

1. Cook the Rice: Rinse the brown basmati rice under cold water until the water runs clear. In a medium saucepan, bring 2 1/2 cups of water to a

boil. Add the rice and a pinch of salt, then reduce the heat to low, cover, and simmer for about 35-40 minutes, or until the water is absorbed and the rice is tender. Remove from heat and let it sit, covered, for 5 minutes.

2. Prepare the Curry: While the rice is cooking, heat the coconut oil in a large pot over medium heat. Add the onion, garlic, and ginger, and sauté until the onion is translucent and soft, about 5 minutes.

3. Add Spices and Squash: Stir in the garam masala, turmeric, cumin, and chili powder, cooking for another minute until fragrant. Add the cubed butternut squash and toss to coat with the spices.

4. Simmer the Curry: Add the chickpeas, coconut milk, and vegetable broth to the pot. Bring the mixture to a boil, then reduce the heat to low, cover, and simmer for about 30 minutes,

or until the butternut squash is tender and the curry has thickened. Season with salt and pepper to taste.

5. Serve: Fluff the cooked rice with a fork. Spoon the curry over a bed of brown basmati rice and garnish with chopped cilantro.

Nutritional Information (per serving):

Calories: 530| Protein: 12g| Carbohydrates: 85g| Fat: 18g| Saturated Fat: 13g| Sodium: 300mg| Fiber: 10g| Sugar: 10g

ZUCCHINI LASAGNA WITH RICOTTA AND SPINACH

This healthy twist on traditional lasagna uses thinly sliced zucchini in place of pasta, layered with a creamy ricotta and spinach filling, topped with marinara sauce and melted cheese. It's a lighter, low-carb option that doesn't skimp on flavor.

Serves: 6 servings| Prep Time: 30 minutes| Cooking Time: 45 minutes| Total Time: 1 hour 15 minutes

Ingredients:

For the Zucchini Layers:

- 4 large zucchinis, sliced lengthwise into thin strips

- 1 tablespoon olive oil

- Salt and pepper, to taste

For the Ricotta Spinach Filling:

- 1 container (15 ounces) ricotta cheese

- 1 egg

- 1/4 cup grated Parmesan cheese

- 2 cups fresh spinach, chopped

- 1 teaspoon garlic powder

- Salt and pepper, to taste

For Assembly:

- 2 cups marinara sauce

- 2 cups shredded mozzarella cheese

- Fresh basil leaves, for garnish (optional)

Instructions:

1. Prep the Zucchini: Set your oven to 375°F (190°C). Brush the zucchini slices with olive oil and season with salt and pepper. Arrange the slices on baking sheets and bake for about 15 minutes to remove excess moisture. Set aside to cool.

2. Prepare the Ricotta Spinach Filling: In a bowl, mix together the ricotta cheese, egg, Parmesan cheese, chopped spinach, garlic powder, salt, and pepper until well combined.

3. Assemble the Lasagna: Spread a thin layer of marinara sauce on the bottom of a 9x13 inch baking dish. Layer zucchini slices to cover the bottom. Spread half of the ricotta mixture over the zucchini and then spoon a layer of marinara sauce over the top. Sprinkle with a third of the mozzarella cheese. Repeat the layers, ending with a layer of zucchini slices. Top with the remaining marinara sauce and mozzarella cheese.

4. Bake: Cover the dish with aluminum foil and bake in the preheated oven for 30 minutes. Remove the foil and bake for an additional 15 minutes, or until the cheese is bubbly and golden. Let the lasagna stand for 10 minutes before slicing.

5. Serve: Garnish with fresh basil leaves before serving, if desired.

Nutritional Information (per serving):

Calories: 350| Protein: 25g| Carbohydrates: 15g| Fat: 20g| Saturated Fat: 10g| Cholesterol: 80mg| Sodium: 700mg| Fiber: 3g| Sugar: 8g

RECIPE 9

ROASTED TURMERIC CAULIFLOWER STEAKS WITH GREEN BEANS

This vibrant and healthy dish features thick slices of cauliflower seasoned with turmeric and roasted to perfection, served alongside crisp green beans. It's a simple yet flavorful meal that's packed with nutrients and suitable for a variety of dietary needs.

Serves: 4 servings| Prep Time: 10 minutes| Cooking Time: 25 minutes| Total Time: 35 minutes

Ingredients:

For the Cauliflower Steaks:

- 2 large heads of cauliflower

- 2 tablespoons olive oil

- 1 teaspoon ground turmeric

- 1/2 teaspoon garlic powder

- Salt and pepper, to taste

For the Green Beans:

- 1 pound green beans, trimmed

- 1 tablespoon olive oil

- Salt and pepper, to taste

- Lemon wedges, for serving

Instructions:

1. Preheat the Oven: Set your oven to 425°F (220°C). Line a baking sheet with parchment paper.

2. Prepare the Cauliflower Steaks: Remove the leaves from the cauliflower and cut off the stem, making sure to keep the core intact. Place the cauliflower on its base and slice into 1-inch thick steaks. You should get about 2-3 steaks per head, depending on the size.

3. Season the Cauliflower: Place the cauliflower steaks on the prepared baking sheet. Brush both sides with olive oil and sprinkle evenly with turmeric, garlic powder, salt, and pepper.

4. Roast the Cauliflower: Bake in the preheated oven for about 20-25 minutes, or until the cauliflower is tender and the edges are golden brown.

5. Prepare the Green Beans: While the cauliflower is roasting, toss the green beans with 1 tablespoon of olive oil, salt, and pepper. Spread them out on another baking sheet.

6. Roast the Green Beans: Add the green beans

to the oven during the last 10 minutes of the cauliflower's cooking time. Roast until they are tender and slightly crisp.

7. Serve: Arrange the cauliflower steaks and green beans on a plate. Serve with lemon wedges on the side for added flavor.

Nutritional Information (per serving):

Calories: 150| Protein: 5g| Carbohydrates: 15g| Fat: 9g| Saturated Fat: 1g| Sodium: 50mg| Fiber: 6g| Sugar: 5g

RECIPE 10

PORTOBELLO MUSHROOM CAPS WITH QUINOA PILAF AND STEAMED KALE

This wholesome dish features juicy Portobello

mushroom caps paired with a flavorful quinoa pilaf and tender steamed kale, making for a nutritious and satisfying meal that's perfect for a healthy dinner option.

Serves: 4 servings| Prep Time: 15 minutes| Cooking Time: 25 minutes| Total Time: 40 minutes

Ingredients:

For the Portobello Mushroom Caps:

- 4 large Portobello mushroom caps, stems removed

- 2 tablespoons olive oil

- 2 cloves garlic, minced

- Salt and pepper, to taste

For the Quinoa Pilaf:

- 1 cup quinoa, rinsed

- 2 cups vegetable broth

- 1 small onion, finely chopped

- 1 carrot, diced

- 1/2 cup frozen peas

- 1 teaspoon dried thyme

- 1 tablespoon olive oil

- Salt and pepper, to taste

For the Steamed Kale:

- 1 bunch kale, stems removed and leaves chopped

- Salt and pepper, to taste

Instructions:

1. Cook the Quinoa Pilaf: In a medium saucepan, heat 1 tablespoon of olive oil over medium heat. Add the onion and carrot, and sauté until softened, about 5 minutes. Add the rinsed quinoa, vegetable broth, dried thyme, and a pinch of salt and pepper. Bring to a boil, then reduce the heat to low, cover, and simmer for 15 minutes, or until the liquid is absorbed and the quinoa is fluffy. Stir in the frozen peas during the last 5 minutes of cooking.

2. Prepare the Portobello Caps: Set your oven to 400°F (200°C). Brush both sides of the Portobello mushroom caps with olive oil and sprinkle with minced garlic, salt, and pepper. Place them gill-side up on a baking sheet.

3. Roast the Mushrooms: Roast the mushroom caps in the preheated oven for about 15-20 minutes, or until they are tender and juicy.

4. Steam the Kale: While the mushrooms are roasting, bring a pot of water to a boil and place a steamer basket with chopped kale over the water. Cover and steam for about 5-7 minutes, or until the kale is tender but still vibrant green. Season with salt and pepper to taste.

5. Serve: Place a Portobello mushroom cap on each plate. Spoon the quinoa pilaf into the caps, allowing some to spill over onto the plate if desired. Serve the steamed kale on the side.

Nutritional Information (per serving):

Calories: 320| Protein: 11g| Carbohydrates: 40g| Fat: 15g| Saturated Fat: 2g| Sodium: 300mg| Fiber: 7g| Sugar: 5g

Dessert Recipes

Recipe 1

Baked Apples with Cinnamon and Nutmeg

This cozy dessert features tender, baked apples filled with a warmly spiced mixture of cinnamon and nutmeg, making it a perfect treat for chilly evenings or any time you crave a comforting sweet.

Serves: 4 servings | Prep Time: 10 minutes | Cooking Time: 30 minutes | Total Time: 40 minutes

Ingredients:

- 4 large apples (such as Granny Smith or Honeycrisp)

- 1/4 cup brown sugar

- 1 teaspoon ground cinnamon

- 1/4 teaspoon ground nutmeg

- 1/4 cup chopped walnuts or pecans (optional)

- 4 teaspoons butter

- 1/2 cup apple cider or water

- Vanilla ice cream or whipped cream, for serving (optional)

Instructions:

1. Preheat the Oven: Set your oven to 375°F (190°C).

2. Prepare the Apples: Core the apples, making a large well in the center and leaving the bottom intact. If necessary, slice a small amount off the bottom of each apple to create a flat surface

so they stand upright.

3. Mix the Filling: In a small bowl, combine the brown sugar, cinnamon, nutmeg, and chopped nuts (if using).

4. Fill the Apples: Spoon the sugar and spice mixture into the wells of the apples, pressing down slightly to pack. Top each apple with a teaspoon of butter.

5. Bake the Apples: Place the apples in a baking dish and pour the apple cider or water into the bottom of the dish. Bake for 30-35 minutes, or until the apples are tender when pierced with a fork.

6. Serve: Allow the apples to cool slightly, then serve warm with the juices spooned over the top. Add a scoop of vanilla ice cream or a dollop of whipped cream, if desired.

Nutritional Information (per serving, without

optional ingredients):

Calories: 180| Protein: 0g| Carbohydrates: 38g| Fat: 4g| Saturated Fat: 2.5g| Sodium: 30mg| Fiber: 5g| Sugar: 31g

RECIPE 2

CHIA SEED PUDDING WITH MIXED BERRY COMPOTE

This nutritious and delicious chia seed pudding is paired with a vibrant mixed berry compote, offering a perfect balance of creamy texture and tart sweetness. It's an ideal breakfast or dessert that's both healthy and satisfying.

Serves: 4 servings | Prep Time: 15 minutes (plus overnight for setting) | Cooking Time: 10 minutes | Total Time: 25 minutes active, plus overnight setting

Ingredients:

For the Chia Pudding:

- 1/4 cup chia seeds

- 1 cup almond milk (or any milk of your choice)

- 1 tablespoon maple syrup or honey

- 1/2 teaspoon vanilla extract

For the Mixed Berry Compote:

- 2 cups mixed berries (fresh or frozen)

- 2 tablespoons maple syrup or honey

- 1 teaspoon lemon juice

- 1/2 teaspoon vanilla extract

Instructions:

1. Prepare the Chia Pudding: In a mixing bowl, combine the chia seeds, almond milk, maple syrup (or honey), and vanilla extract. Stir well to mix. Let the mixture sit for 5 minutes, then stir again to break up any clumps. Cover and refrigerate overnight, or for at least 6 hours, until the pudding has thickened and the chia seeds have absorbed the liquid.

2. Make the Mixed Berry Compote: In a small saucepan, combine the mixed berries, maple syrup (or honey), and lemon juice. Cook over medium heat, stirring occasionally, until the berries have softened and released their juices, about 5-10 minutes. Remove from heat and stir in the vanilla extract. Let the compote cool slightly, then refrigerate until ready to use.

3. Assemble the Puddings: Give the chia pudding a good stir to ensure a smooth texture. Spoon the chia pudding into serving glasses or bowls. Top with the chilled mixed berry compote.

4. Serve: Enjoy the chia seed pudding with mixed berry compote immediately, or keep refrigerated until ready to serve. Can be enjoyed cold from the fridge.

Nutritional Information (per serving):

Calories: 180| Protein: 4g| Carbohydrates: 29g| Fat: 6g| Saturated Fat: 0.5g| Sodium: 45mg| Fiber: 8g| Sugar: 18g

CARROT AND WALNUT MUFFINS SWEETENED WITH APPLE SAUCE

These moist and flavorful muffins are a healthier treat, using apple sauce as a natural sweetener and incorporating the goodness of carrots and walnuts. They're perfect for breakfast, a snack, or even a light dessert.

Serves: 12 muffins| Prep Time: 15 minutes| Cooking Time: 20 minutes| Total Time: 35 minutes

Ingredients:

- 1 1/2 cups whole wheat flour

- 1 teaspoon baking soda

- 1 1/2 teaspoons ground cinnamon

- 1/2 teaspoon ground nutmeg

- 1/4 teaspoon salt

- 3/4 cup unsweetened apple sauce

- 1/2 cup vegetable oil

- 2 large eggs

- 1 teaspoon vanilla extract

- 1 1/2 cups grated carrots (about 2-3 medium carrots)

- 1/2 cup chopped walnuts

- 1/4 cup raisins (optional)

Instructions:

1. Preheat the Oven and Prep the Muffin Tin: Set your oven to 350°F (175°C). Line a 12-cup

muffin tin with paper liners or lightly grease the cups.

2. Mix Dry Ingredients: In a large bowl, whisk together the whole wheat flour, baking soda, cinnamon, nutmeg, and salt.

3. Combine Wet Ingredients: In a separate bowl, mix the apple sauce, vegetable oil, eggs, and vanilla extract until well combined.

4. Combine Wet and Dry Mixtures: Add the wet ingredients to the dry ingredients, stirring just until combined. Avoid overmixing to keep the muffins light and fluffy.

5. Add Carrots, Walnuts, and Raisins: Fold in the grated carrots, chopped walnuts, and raisins (if using) until evenly distributed throughout the batter.

6. Fill Muffin Cups and Bake: Divide the batter evenly among the prepared muffin cups, filling

each about 3/4 full. Bake for 20-25 minutes, or until a toothpick inserted into the center of a muffin comes out clean.

7. Cool and Serve: Allow the muffins to cool in the pan for 5 minutes, then transfer them to a wire rack to cool completely. Serve warm or at room temperature.

Nutritional Information (per muffin):

Calories: 200| Protein: 4g| Carbohydrates: 24g| Fat: 11g| Saturated Fat: 1.5g| Cholesterol: 30mg| Sodium: 150mg| Fiber: 3g| Sugar: 8g

Carrot and Walnut Muffins Sweetened with Apple Sauce offer a delightful way to enjoy a healthier treat. Packed with the goodness of whole grains, fruits, and vegetables, these muffins are sure to satisfy your sweet tooth in a more nutritious way.

RECIPE 4

AVOCADO CHOCOLATE MOUSSE

This rich and creamy avocado chocolate mousse is a healthier alternative to traditional mousse, using ripe avocados for a silky texture and natural sweetness. It's a decadent yet nutritious dessert that's sure to satisfy chocolate cravings.

Serves: 4 servings| Prep Time: 10 minutes| Cooking Time: 0 minutes (chill for at least 1 hour) | Total Time: 1 hour 10 minutes

Ingredients:

- 2 ripe avocados, pitted and scooped

- 1/4 cup cocoa powder, unsweetened

- 1/4 cup honey or maple syrup (adjust to taste)

- 1/2 teaspoon vanilla extract

- A pinch of salt

- 2-4 tablespoons milk (any kind), as needed for consistency

- Fresh berries or whipped cream, for garnish (optional)

Instructions:

1. Blend the Ingredients: In a food processor or high-speed blender, combine the scooped avocado, cocoa powder, honey (or maple syrup), vanilla extract, and a pinch of salt. Blend until smooth and creamy.

2. Adjust Consistency and Taste: If the mixture

is too thick, add milk, one tablespoon at a time, until you reach your desired consistency. Taste the mousse and adjust the sweetness if needed by adding a bit more honey or maple syrup.

3. Chill the Mousse: Transfer the mousse to individual serving dishes or a large bowl. Cover and refrigerate for at least 1 hour to allow the flavors to meld together and the mousse to set.

4. Serve: Once chilled, garnish the avocado chocolate mousse with fresh berries, whipped cream, or a sprinkle of cocoa powder before serving.

Nutritional Information (per serving):

Calories: 250| Protein: 3g| Carbohydrates: 30g| Fat: 15g| Saturated Fat: 2.5g| Sodium: 30mg| Fiber: 7g| Sugar: 20g

ALMOND AND DATE ENERGY BALLS

These no-bake almond and date energy balls are a perfect healthy snack, packed with natural sweetness from dates and the nutty crunch of almonds. They're easy to make, require no cooking, and are ideal for a quick energy boost.

Serves: Makes about 12 balls | Prep Time: 15 minutes | Cooking Time: 0 minutes | Total Time: 15 minutes (plus time for chilling, if preferred)

Ingredients:

- 1 cup Medjool dates, pitted (about 10-12

dates)

- 1 cup raw almonds

- 1/2 cup shredded unsweetened coconut

- 1 tablespoon chia seeds (optional)

- 1 teaspoon vanilla extract

- A pinch of salt

- 2 tablespoons water, if needed for blending

Instructions:

1. Process Dates and Almonds: In a food processor, combine the pitted dates and raw almonds. Pulse until they are finely chopped and the mixture starts to clump together.

2. Add Remaining Ingredients: Add the shredded coconut, chia seeds (if using), vanilla extract, and a pinch of salt to the food processor. Pulse

several times until all ingredients are well combined. If the mixture is too dry to form into balls, add water, one tablespoon at a time, until it reaches the desired consistency.

3. Form the Energy Balls: Using your hands, roll the mixture into small balls, about the size of a walnut. If the mixture is sticky, wetting your hands slightly can help prevent sticking.

4. Chill (Optional): While these energy balls can be eaten right away, chilling them in the refrigerator for an hour can enhance their texture and flavor.

5. Serve or Store: Serve the energy balls immediately, or store them in an airtight container in the refrigerator for up to a week, or in the freezer for a longer shelf life.

Nutritional Information (per ball, if 12 made):

Calories: 150| Protein: 4g| Carbohydrates: 18g| Fat: 8g| Saturated Fat: 2g| Sodium: 20mg| Fiber: 4g| Sugar: 13g

RECIPE 6

COCONUT YOGURT WITH FRESH MANGO AND TOASTED COCONUT FLAKES

This refreshing and tropical-inspired breakfast or snack features creamy coconut yogurt topped with juicy fresh mango and crunchy toasted coconut flakes. It's a delightful combination of flavors and textures, perfect for a nutritious start to your day or a light dessert.

Serves: 4 servings| Prep Time: 10 minutes| Cooking Time: 0 minutes (plus 5 minutes if toasting coconut flakes)| Total Time: 10

minutes (plus 5 minutes if toasting coconut flakes)

Ingredients:

- 2 cups coconut yogurt

- 2 ripe mangoes, peeled and diced

- 1/2 cup coconut flakes

- Optional: honey or maple syrup for drizzling, mint leaves for garnish

Instructions:

1. Toast the Coconut Flakes: In a dry skillet over medium heat, toast the coconut flakes, stirring frequently, until they're golden brown and fragrant. This should take about 3-5 minutes. Remove from heat and allow to cool.

2. Prepare the Mango: Peel and dice the mangoes into bite-sized pieces.

3. Assemble the Bowls: Divide the coconut yogurt among four serving bowls. Top each bowl with an equal amount of diced mango.

4. Add Toppings: Sprinkle the toasted coconut flakes over each serving. If desired, drizzle with a little honey or maple syrup for added sweetness and garnish with mint leaves.

5. Serve: Enjoy this coconut yogurt with fresh mango and toasted coconut flakes immediately for the best combination of textures and flavors.

Nutritional Information (per serving):

Calories: 250 | Protein: 5g | Carbohydrates: 35g | Fat: 11g | Saturated Fat: 9g | Sodium: 35mg | Fiber: 5g | Sugar: 30g

RECIPE 7

ROASTED PEAR WITH HONEY AND WALNUTS

This elegant and simple dessert features ripe pears roasted to perfection, then drizzled with honey and sprinkled with crunchy walnuts. It's a warm, comforting dish that perfectly balances sweetness and texture, ideal for a cozy evening or to impress guests.

Serves: 4 servings| Prep Time: 10 minutes| Cooking Time: 25 minutes| Total Time: 35 minutes

Ingredients:

- 4 ripe but firm pears, halved and cored

- 2 tablespoons unsalted butter, melted

- 4 tablespoons honey, plus more for drizzling

- 1/2 cup walnuts, roughly chopped

- A pinch of ground cinnamon (optional)

- Vanilla ice cream or whipped cream, for serving (optional)

Instructions:

1. Preheat the Oven: Set your oven to 375°F (190°C).

2. Prepare the Pears: After halving and coring the pears, place them cut-side up on a baking

dish. Brush the pears with melted butter, ensuring the cut surfaces are well coated.

3. Add Honey and Walnuts: Drizzle each pear half with about 1/2 tablespoon of honey. Sprinkle the chopped walnuts over the top, and if desired, add a pinch of cinnamon for extra flavor.

4. Roast the Pears: Place the baking dish in the preheated oven and roast the pears for about 25 minutes, or until they are tender and the walnuts are toasted.

5. Serve: Once the pears are roasted, allow them to cool slightly. Serve each pear half with a drizzle of honey and, if desired, a scoop of vanilla ice cream or a dollop of whipped cream.

Nutritional Information (per serving):

Calories: 270| Protein: 3g| Carbohydrates:

38g| Fat: 14g| Saturated Fat: 4g| Cholesterol: 15mg| Sodium: 5mg| Fiber: 6g| Sugar: 28g

RECIPE 8

NO-BAKE OATMEAL AND PEANUT BUTTER BARS

These no-bake oatmeal and peanut butter bars are a quick, easy, and delicious snack. Packed with the wholesome goodness of oats and the creamy richness of peanut butter, they're perfect for a healthy treat on the go.

Serves: 12 bars| Prep Time:15 minutes| Setting Time: 1 hour in the refrigerator| Total Time: 1

hour 15 minutes

Ingredients:

- 2 cups rolled oats

- 1 cup natural peanut butter (smooth or crunchy, according to preference)

- 1/2 cup honey or maple syrup

- 1/2 cup mini chocolate chips (optional)

- 1 teaspoon vanilla extract

- A pinch of salt

Instructions:

1. Mix the Ingredients: In a large mixing bowl, combine the rolled oats, peanut butter, honey (or maple syrup), vanilla extract, and a pinch of

salt. Stir well until all the ingredients are thoroughly mixed. If the mixture seems too dry, add a little more peanut butter or honey to reach a sticky consistency.

2. Add Chocolate Chips: Gently fold in the mini chocolate chips, if using, ensuring they're evenly distributed throughout the mixture.

3. Press into a Pan: Line an 8x8 inch (20x20 cm) square baking pan with parchment paper, leaving some overhang on the sides for easy removal. Transfer the oat mixture to the pan and press it down firmly and evenly with the back of a spoon or your hands.

4. Chill: Place the pan in the refrigerator and let the mixture set for at least 1 hour, until firm.

5. Cut into Bars: Once set, use the parchment paper overhang to lift the mixture out of the pan. Place it on a cutting board and cut into 12 equal bars.

6. Serve or Store: Enjoy the oatmeal and peanut butter bars immediately, or store them in an airtight container in the refrigerator for up to a week.

Nutritional Information (per bar):

Calories: 230| Protein: 6g| Carbohydrates: 27g| Fat: 12g| Saturated Fat: 2.5g| Sodium: 100mg| Fiber: 3g| Sugar: 15g

RECIPE 9

RASPBERRY AND LEMON SORBET

This refreshing raspberry and lemon sorbet is a perfect palate cleanser or a light dessert for a warm day. With just a few ingredients, you can create a vibrant, tangy treat that's both easy to make and delightfully delicious.

Serves: 6 servings| Prep Time:| 10 minutes| Freezing Time: 2 hours or until firm| Total Time: 2 hours 10 minutes

Ingredients:

- 4 cups fresh raspberries

- 3/4 cup sugar (adjust based on sweetness of raspberries and personal preference)

- 1 cup water

- 1/2 cup freshly squeezed lemon juice (about 2 -3 lemons)

- Lemon zest from 1 lemon (optional for added flavor)

Instructions:

1. Make the Simple Syrup: In a small saucepan, combine the sugar and water. Heat over medium heat, stirring until the sugar has completely dissolved. Remove from heat and let cool to

room temperature.

2. Blend the Raspberries: In a blender or food processor, puree the raspberries until smooth. If desired, strain the puree through a fine-mesh sieve to remove seeds, but this step is optional.

3. Combine and Chill: Mix the raspberry puree, cooled simple syrup, lemon juice, and lemon zest (if using) in a large bowl. Stir until well combined. Cover and chill the mixture in the refrigerator for about 1 hour, or until it's cold.

4. Churn the Sorbet: Pour the chilled mixture into an ice cream maker and churn according to the manufacturer's instructions, until it reaches a smooth, sorbet consistency.

5. Freeze to Firm Up: Transfer the sorbet to a freezer-safe container, cover, and freeze until firm, at least 2 hours or overnight.

6. Serve: Scoop the sorbet into bowls or

glasses. If desired, garnish with fresh raspberries or a twist of lemon zest before serving.

Nutritional Information (per serving):

Calories: 130| Protein: 1g| Carbohydrates: 34g| Fat: 0g| Saturated Fat: 0g| Sodium: 0mg| Fiber: 4g| Sugar: 29g

RECIPE 10

BAKED PEACH HALVES WITH CINNAMON AND ALMOND CRUMBLE

This delicious dessert features juicy baked peaches topped with a crunchy cinnamon and almond crumble, a perfect blend of sweetness and texture. It's a simple, comforting dish ideal for summer evenings or whenever you have ripe peaches on hand.

Serves: 6 servings | Prep Time: 15 minute |
Cooking Time: 25 minutes | Total Time: 40
minutes

Ingredients:

For the Peaches:

- 6 ripe peaches, halved and pitted

- 2 tablespoons honey or maple syrup

- 1/2 teaspoon ground cinnamon

For the Almond Crumble:

- 1/2 cup rolled oats

- 1/2 cup almond flour

- 1/4 cup sliced almonds

- 1/4 cup unsalted butter, melted

- 1/4 cup brown sugar

- 1/2 teaspoon ground cinnamon

- A pinch of salt

Instructions:

1. Preheat the Oven: Set your oven to 375°F (190°C). Arrange the peach halves, cut side up, in a baking dish.

2. Prepare the Peaches: Drizzle honey (or maple syrup) over the peach halves and sprinkle with ground cinnamon.

3. Make the Almond Crumble: In a mixing bowl, combine the rolled oats, almond flour, sliced almonds, melted butter, brown sugar, cinnamon, and a pinch of salt. Mix until the ingredients are well combined and the mixture resembles a coarse crumble.

4. Top the Peaches: Spoon the almond crumble

mixture over the peach halves, pressing it lightly to adhere.

5. Bake: Place the baking dish in the preheated oven and bake for 25 minutes, or until the peaches are tender and the crumble is golden brown and crisp.

6. Serve: Allow the baked peaches to cool slightly before serving. They can be enjoyed on their own or with a dollop of vanilla ice cream or whipped cream for an extra indulgent touch.

Nutritional Information (per serving):

Calories: 280| Protein: 5g| Carbohydrates: 38g| Fat: 14g| Saturated Fat: 5g| Sodium: 10mg| Fiber: 5g| Sugar: 29g

SMOOTHIES RECIPES

RECIPE 1

GREEN DETOX SMOOTHIE WITH SPINACH, KIWI, AND GINGER

This revitalizing Green Detox Smoothie is packed with spinach, kiwi, and ginger, making it a perfect blend of nutrients and flavors. It's ideal for a refreshing start to your day or a nourishing mid-day boost.

Serves: 2 servings | Prep Time: 10 minutes | Cooking Time: 0 minutes | Total Time: 10 minutes

Ingredients:

- 2 cups fresh spinach leaves, washed

- 2 ripe kiwis, peeled and sliced

- 1 small piece of fresh ginger (about 1 inch), peeled and grated

- 1 banana, sliced and frozen (for creaminess and chill)

- 1 cup unsweetened almond milk (or any milk of your choice)

- 1 tablespoon chia seeds (optional for extra fiber and omega-3s)

- Juice of 1/2 lemon

- Ice cubes (optional, for extra chill)

- Honey or maple syrup to taste (optional, for added sweetness)

Instructions:

1. Prepare Ingredients: Ensure all fruits are

properly washed, peeled, and sliced as needed. For the ginger, use a spoon to peel the skin off before grating.

2. Blend the Smoothie: In a high-speed blender, combine the spinach, kiwi slices, grated ginger, frozen banana, almond milk, chia seeds (if using), and lemon juice. Blend on high until the mixture is smooth and creamy. If the smoothie is too thick, you can add a little more almond milk to reach your desired consistency.

3. Adjust Taste: Taste the smoothie and, if desired, add honey or maple syrup to sweeten it to your liking. Blend again briefly to mix in the sweetener if you've added it.

4. Serve: Pour the smoothie into glasses. If you prefer a colder drink, blend with a few ice cubes or serve over ice. Enjoy immediately for the best flavor and nutrient content.

Nutritional Information (per serving):

Calories: 180| Protein: 4g| Carbohydrates: 35g| Fat: 3g| Saturated Fat: 0g| Sodium: 95mg| Fiber: 7g| Sugar: 20g (varies depending on the use of sweetener)

RECIPE 2

BERRY ANTIOXIDANT SMOOTHIE WITH BLUEBERRIES, RASPBERRIES, AND FLAXSEED

This Berry Antioxidant Smoothie is a delicious blend of blueberries, raspberries, and flaxseed, offering a powerful dose of antioxidants and essential nutrients. It's perfect for a nutritious breakfast or a refreshing snack.

Serves: 2 servings| Prep Time: 10 minutes| Cooking Time: 0 minutes| Total Time: 10 minutes

Ingredients:

- 1 cup blueberries (fresh or frozen)

- 1 cup raspberries (fresh or frozen)

- 1 banana, sliced and frozen

- 2 tablespoons ground flaxseed

- 1 cup spinach leaves (optional for extra nutrients)

- 1 cup unsweetened almond milk (or any milk of your choice)

- Ice cubes (optional, if you prefer a colder smoothie)

- Honey or maple syrup to taste (optional, for added sweetness)

Instructions:

1. Prepare the Ingredients: If you're using fresh berries, wash them thoroughly. If you're using frozen berries, they're ready to go directly into the blender. Ensure the banana is sliced and frozen ahead of time for a creamier texture.

2. Blend the Smoothie: In a blender, combine the blueberries, raspberries, frozen banana slices, ground flaxseed, and spinach leaves (if using). Add the almond milk and blend on high until the mixture is smooth and creamy. If the smoothie is thicker than you prefer, you can add a little more milk to adjust the consistency.

3. Adjust Consistency and Sweetness: If you're

using fresh berries and prefer a colder smoothie, add a few ice cubes and blend again. Taste the smoothie and, if desired, add honey or maple syrup to sweeten it to your liking, then blend briefly to incorporate the sweetener.

4. Serve: Pour the smoothie into glasses and serve immediately. You can garnish with a few whole berries or a sprinkle of ground flaxseed on top for presentation.

Nutritional Information (per serving):

Calories: 190| Protein: 4g| Carbohydrates: 37g| Fat: 4.5g| Saturated Fat: 0.5g| Sodium: 95mg| Fiber: 11g| Sugar: 20g (varies depending on the use of sweetener and the sweetness of the berries)

PROTEIN POWER SMOOTHIE WITH ALMOND BUTTER, BANANA, AND HEMP SEEDS

This Protein Power Smoothie blends almond butter, banana, and hemp seeds for a creamy, nutrient-rich drink that's perfect for a post-workout refuel or a substantial breakfast. It's packed with protein, healthy fats, and essential nutrients to keep you energized.

Serves: 2 servings | Prep Time: 5 minutes | Cooking Time: 0 minutes | Total Time: 5 minutes

Ingredients:

- 2 ripe bananas, sliced and frozen

- 2 tablespoons almond butter

- 2 tablespoons hemp seeds

- 1 cup unsweetened almond milk (or any milk of your choice)

- 1 scoop protein powder (optional, for an extra protein boost)

- 1 teaspoon vanilla extract

- Ice cubes (optional, for added thickness)

- Honey or maple syrup to taste (optional, for added sweetness)

Instructions:

1. Prepare the Ingredients: Ensure the bananas are peeled, sliced, and frozen ahead of time. Measure out the almond butter, hemp seeds, and any other ingredients you'll be using.

2. Blend the Smoothie: In a high-speed blender, combine the frozen banana slices, almond butter, hemp seeds, almond milk, protein powder (if using), and vanilla extract. Blend on high until the mixture is smooth and creamy.

3. Adjust Consistency and Taste: If the smoothie is too thick, you can add more almond milk to achieve your desired consistency. If you prefer a sweeter smoothie, add honey or maple syrup to taste, then blend again to mix.

4. Serve: Pour the smoothie into glasses. If desired, you can sprinkle a few hemp seeds on top or slice a bit of banana for garnish.

Nutritional Information (per serving, without optional ingredients):

Calories: 280| Protein: 10g| Carbohydrates: 30g| Fat: 16g| Saturated Fat: 1.5g| Sodium: 95mg| Fiber: 6g| Sugar: 14g

TROPICAL IMMUNE BOOSTER SMOOTHIE WITH PINEAPPLE, MANGO, AND TURMERIC

This vibrant Tropical Immune Booster Smoothie combines pineapple, mango, and turmeric for a deliciously sweet and spicy blend. It's packed with vitamins, antioxidants, and anti-inflammatory properties, making it a perfect drink for boosting your immune system and refreshing your palate.

Serves: 2 servings| Prep Time: 10 minutes| Cooking Time: 0 minutes| Total Time: 10 minutes

Ingredients:

- 1 cup fresh or frozen pineapple chunks

- 1 cup fresh or frozen mango chunks

- 1 small piece of fresh turmeric root (about 1 inch), peeled and grated (or 1/2 teaspoon ground turmeric)

- 1 banana, sliced and frozen

- 1 cup coconut water or regular water (adjust according to desired consistency)

- Juice of 1 lime

- A pinch of black pepper (to enhance turmeric absorption)

- Optional: 1 tablespoon honey or agave syrup for added sweetness

- Optional: 1 scoop of protein powder or a handful of spinach for an extra nutrient boost

Instructions:

1. Prepare Ingredients: If using fresh fruits, peel, and cut them into chunks. If using frozen, they're ready to go. Peel and grate the turmeric root, if using fresh.

2. Blend the Smoothie: In a blender, combine the pineapple chunks, mango chunks, grated turmeric (or ground turmeric), frozen banana slices, coconut water, and lime juice. Blend on high until the mixture is smooth and creamy. If the smoothie is too thick, add a little more coconut water until you reach your desired consistency.

3. Enhance Absorption: Add a pinch of black pepper to the smoothie and blend again for a few seconds. Black pepper contains piperine, which can significantly boost the absorption of curcumin, the active ingredient in turmeric.

4. Adjust Taste: Taste the smoothie, and if you prefer it sweeter, add honey or agave syrup, then blend again to mix.

5. Serve: Pour the smoothie into glasses and serve immediately. Enjoy the tropical flavors and the immune-boosting benefits!

Nutritional Information (per serving, without optional ingredients):

Calories: 160| Protein: 2g|Carbohydrates: 40g| Fat: 0.5g| Saturated Fat: 0g| Sodium: 125mg| Fiber: 5g| Sugar: 30g

RECIPE 5

HEART-HEALTHY AVOCADO AND CACAO SMOOTHIE

This Heart-Healthy Avocado and Cacao Smoothie combines the creamy texture of avocado with the rich flavor of cacao, creating a deliciously indulgent yet nutritious drink. Packed with healthy fats, fiber, and antioxidants, it's perfect for a heart-friendly breakfast or a satisfying snack.

Serves: 2 servings | Prep Time: 5 minutes | Cooking Time: 0 minutes | Total Time: 5 minutes

Ingredients:

- 1 ripe avocado, pitted and scooped

- 2 tablespoons raw cacao powder (or unsweetened cocoa powder)

- 1 banana, sliced and frozen

- 1 cup almond milk (or any milk of your choice)

- 1 tablespoon chia seeds

- 1 tablespoon honey or maple syrup (adjust to taste)

- A pinch of sea salt

- Ice cubes (optional, for a thicker smoothie)

Instructions:

1. Blend Ingredients: In a blender, combine the avocado, cacao powder, frozen banana slices, almond milk, chia seeds, honey (or maple syrup), and a pinch of sea salt. Blend on high until the mixture becomes smooth and creamy.

2. Adjust Consistency: If the smoothie is too thick, add a little more almond milk and blend again. For a colder, thicker smoothie, add a few ice cubes and blend to your desired consistency.

3. Taste and Sweeten: Taste the smoothie and, if desired, add more honey or maple syrup to

sweeten it further. Blend briefly to incorporate any additional sweetener.

4. Serve: Pour the smoothie into glasses and serve immediately. Enjoy the rich, creamy texture and the heart-healthy benefits!

Nutritional Information (per serving):

Calories: 290| Protein: 5g| Carbohydrates: 36g| Fat: 17g| Saturated Fat: 2.5g| Sodium: 95mg| Fiber: 13g| Sugar: 17g

RECIPE 6

PEACH AND OAT BREAKFAST

SMOOTHIE

This Peach and Oat Breakfast Smoothie is a hearty and delicious way to start your day. Combining the natural sweetness of peaches with the filling texture of oats, this smoothie is both nutritious and satisfying, making it an ideal breakfast on the go.

Serves: 2 servings| Prep Time: 10 minutes| Cooking Time: 0 minutes| Total Time: 10 minutes

Ingredients:

- 2 ripe peaches, pitted and sliced (fresh or frozen)

- 1/2 cup rolled oats

- 1 banana, sliced and frozen

- 1 cup almond milk (or any milk of your choice)

- 1/2 teaspoon vanilla extract

- 1 tablespoon honey or maple syrup (optional, for added sweetness)

- A pinch of cinnamon (optional, for flavor)

- Ice cubes (optional, for a thicker smoothie)

Instructions:

1. Soak the Oats: If you have time, soak the rolled oats in the almond milk for about 10-15 minutes before blending. This can help make the smoothie creamier and the oats easier to digest.

2. Blend the Smoothie: In a blender, combine the soaked oats and milk, peach slices, frozen banana, vanilla extract, and a pinch of cinnamon if using. Blend on high until the mixture is smooth and creamy.

3. Adjust Consistency and TasteIf the smoothie is too thick, add a little more almond milk to achieve your desired consistency. If you prefer a colder smoothie, add a few ice cubes and blend again. Taste the smoothie and, if desired, add honey or maple syrup to sweeten it further, then blend briefly to mix.

4. Serve: Pour the smoothie into glasses and enjoy immediately. You can garnish with a few peach slices or a sprinkle of cinnamon on top for presentation.

Nutritional Information (per serving):

Calories: 220| Protein: 5g| Carbohydrates: 46g| Fat: 3g| Saturated Fat: 0g| Sodium: 95mg| Fiber: 6g| Sugar: 24g

CARROT CAKE SMOOTHIE WITH CARROTS, WALNUTS, AND CINNAMON

This Carrot Cake Smoothie captures all the flavors of the classic dessert in a nutritious and delicious drink. With fresh carrots, walnuts, and cinnamon, it's a wholesome way to enjoy the taste of carrot cake any time of the day without the guilt.

Serves: 2 servings| Prep Time: 10 minutes| Cooking Time: 0 minutes| Total Time: 10 minutes

Ingredients:

- 2 medium carrots, peeled and chopped

- 1 banana, sliced and frozen

- 1/4 cup walnuts

- 1/2 teaspoon ground cinnamon

- 1/4 teaspoon ground nutmeg

- 1 cup unsweetened almond milk (or any milk of your choice)

- 1 tablespoon maple syrup or honey (optional, for added sweetness)

- 1 teaspoon vanilla extract

- 1/2 cup Greek yogurt or coconut yogurt (for creaminess)

- Ice cubes (optional, for a colder smoothie)

Instructions:

1. Prepare the Ingredients: Peel and chop the

carrots into small pieces to ensure they blend smoothly. Slice and freeze the banana ahead of time for a creamier texture.

2. Blend the Smoothie: In a high-speed blender, combine the chopped carrots, frozen banana slices, walnuts, cinnamon, nutmeg, almond milk, vanilla extract, and Greek or coconut yogurt. Blend on high until the mixture is smooth and creamy.

3. Adjust Consistency and Taste: If the smoothie is too thick, add a little more almond milk to achieve your desired consistency. If you prefer a colder smoothie, add a few ice cubes and blend again. Taste the smoothie and, if desired, add maple syrup or honey to sweeten it further, then blend briefly to mix.

4. Serve: Pour the smoothie into glasses and serve immediately. You can garnish with a sprinkle of cinnamon or a few walnut pieces on

top for presentation.

Nutritional Information (per serving):

Calories: 240 | Protein: 8g | Carbohydrates: 30g | Fat: 11g | Saturated Fat: 1.5g | Sodium: 125mg | Fiber: 5g | Sugar: 18g

RECIPE 8

POMEGRANATE AND BEETROOT SMOOTHIE FOR HEART HEALTH

This Pomegranate and Beetroot Smoothie is not only visually stunning but also packed with nutrients beneficial for heart health. The combination of pomegranate and beetroot provides antioxidants, nitrates, and fiber, making this smoothie a powerful drink for supporting cardiovascular wellness.

Serves: 2 servings| Prep Time: 10 minutes| Cooking Time: 0 minutes| Total Time: 10 minutes

Ingredients:

- 1 medium beetroot, cooked and peeled (or raw if you have a high-powered blender)

- 1 cup pomegranate seeds (fresh or frozen)

- 1 banana, sliced and frozen

- 1/2 cup orange juice (freshly squeezed for the best taste)

- 1/2 cup unsweetened almond milk (or any milk of your choice)

- 1 tablespoon chia seeds (optional, for added fiber and omega-3 fatty acids)

- Ice cubes (optional, for a colder smoothie)

Instructions:

1. Prepare Ingredients: If using cooked beetroot, ensure it's cooled and peeled. For a raw beetroot, peel and chop it into smaller pieces. Freeze the banana slices ahead of time for a creamier texture.

2. Blend the Smoothie: In a blender, combine the beetroot, pomegranate seeds, frozen banana slices, orange juice, almond milk, and chia seeds (if using). Blend on high until the mixture is smooth and creamy. If your blender struggles with the beetroot or pomegranate seeds, strain the smoothie through a fine mesh to remove any bits.

3. Adjust Consistency: If the smoothie is too thick, add a little more almond milk or orange juice to achieve your desired consistency. For a colder smoothie, add a few ice cubes and blend

again.

4. Serve: Pour the smoothie into glasses. You can garnish with a few pomegranate seeds or a thin slice of beetroot on the rim of the glass for a decorative touch.

Nutritional Information (per serving):

Calories: 180| Protein: 3g| Carbohydrates: 38g| Fat: 2g| Saturated Fat: 0g| Sodium: 85mg| Fiber: 7g| Sugar: 26g

RECIPE 9

ALMOND JOY SMOOTHIE WITH

ALMONDS, COCONUT, AND DARK CHOCOLATE

This Almond Joy Smoothie captures the essence of the beloved candy bar in a healthier, drinkable form. Combining the flavors of almonds, coconut, and dark chocolate, it's a delicious treat that satisfies sweet cravings while providing nutritional benefits.

Serves: 2 servings| Prep Time: 10 minutes| Cooking Time: 0 minutes| Total Time: 10 minutes

Ingredients:

- 1 banana, sliced and frozen

- 2 tablespoons almond butter

- 1/4 cup unsweetened shredded coconut

- 2 tablespoons dark chocolate chips or cocoa nibs

- 1 cup unsweetened almond milk (or any milk of your choice)

- 1/2 teaspoon vanilla extract

- Ice cubes (optional, for a thicker smoothie)

- Optional toppings: extra shredded coconut, almond slices, and chocolate chips for garnish

Instructions:

1. Prepare Ingredients: Ensure the banana is sliced and frozen ahead of time for a creamier texture. Measure out the almond butter, shredded coconut, and dark chocolate chips or cocoa nibs.

2. Blend the Smoothie: In a blender, combine the frozen banana slices, almond butter,

shredded coconut, dark chocolate chips (or cocoa nibs), almond milk, and vanilla extract. Blend on high until the mixture is smooth and creamy.

3. Adjust Consistency: If the smoothie is too thick, add a little more almond milk and blend again. For a colder, thicker smoothie, add a few ice cubes and blend to your desired consistency.

4. Serve: Pour the smoothie into glasses. If desired, garnish with a sprinkle of shredded coconut, a few almond slices, and some chocolate chips for an extra touch of Almond Joy flavor.

Nutritional Information (per serving):

Calories: 300| Protein: 6g| Carbohydrates: 24g| Fat: 22g| Saturated Fat: 8g| Sodium: 95mg| Fiber: 6g| Sugar: 14g

RECIPE 10

GINGER PEAR SMOOTHIE FOR DIGESTIVE HEALTH

This Ginger Pear Smoothie is designed to support digestive health, blending the soothing properties of ginger with the sweet, refreshing taste of pears. It's a delicious way to aid digestion and enjoy a nutrient-rich treat.

Serves: 2 servings | Prep Time: 10 minutes | Cooking Time: 0 minutes | Total Time: 10 minutes

Ingredients:

- 2 ripe pears, cored and chopped (skin on for

extra fiber)

- 1 small piece of fresh ginger (about 1 inch), peeled and grated

- 1 banana, sliced and frozen

- 1 cup spinach leaves (optional for added nutrients)

- 1 tablespoon ground flaxseed (for omega-3 fatty acids and fiber)

- 1 cup unsweetened almond milk (or any milk of your choice)

- Ice cubes (optional, for a colder smoothie)

- A squeeze of lemon juice (optional, for a tangy flavor)

Instructions:

1. Prepare Ingredients: Wash the pears and

chop them into chunks, keeping the skin on for added fiber. Peel and grate the ginger, and ensure the banana is sliced and frozen.

2. Blend the Smoothie: In a blender, combine the chopped pears, grated ginger, frozen banana slices, spinach leaves (if using), ground flaxseed, and almond milk. Blend on high until the mixture is smooth and creamy.

3. Adjust Consistency and Flavor: If the smoothie is too thick, add a little more almond milk to reach your desired consistency. For a colder smoothie, add a few ice cubes and blend again. Add a squeeze of lemon juice for a tangy kick, if desired.

4. Serve: Pour the smoothie into glasses and enjoy immediately. The combination of ginger and pear not only tastes great but also helps soothe and support digestive health.

Nutritional Information (per serving):

Calories: 190| Protein: 3g| Carbohydrates: 42g| - Fat: 3g| Saturated Fat: 0g| Sodium: 95mg| Fiber: 8g| Sugar: 28g

30 DAYS MEAL PLAN

Week 1:

Day 1:

- **Breakfast**: Avocado and Egg Toast

- **Lunch**: Turmeric Cauliflower Soup with Whole Grain Bread

- **Dinner**: Baked Cod with Lemon Herb Crust and Roasted Asparagus

- **Snacks**: Roasted Red Pepper and Walnut Dip with Whole Wheat Pita Chips (Appetizer), Green Detox Smoothie with Spinach, Kiwi, and Ginger (Smoothie), Baked Apples with Cinnamon and Nutmeg (Dessert)

Day 2:

- **Breakfast**: Greek Yogurt Parfait with Mixed

Berries and Almonds

- **Lunch**: Stuffed Bell Peppers with Quinoa, Black Beans, and Corn

- **Dinner**: Moroccan Lentil and Sweet Potato Stew

- **Snacks**: Cucumber and Hummus Bites (Appetizer), Berry Antioxidant Smoothie with Blueberries, Raspberries, and Flaxseed (Smoothie), Chia Seed Pudding with Mixed Berry Compote (Dessert)

Day 3:

- **Breakfast**: Oatmeal with Sliced Apple, Cinnamon, and Walnuts

- **Lunch**: Beetroot and Goat Cheese Arugula Salad

- **Dinner**: Stuffed Acorn Squash with Wild Rice and Cranberries

- **Snacks**: Zucchini and Carrot Fritters (Appetizer), Protein Power Smoothie with Almond Butter, Banana, and Hemp Seeds (Smoothie), Carrot and Walnut Muffins Sweetened with Apple Sauce (Dessert)

Day 4:

- **Breakfast**: Smoothie Bowl with Spinach, Banana, and Flaxseeds, topped with Pumpkin Seeds

- **Lunch**: Asian-style Tofu Stir-fry with Brown Rice and Mixed Vegetables

- **Dinner**: Grilled Eggplant and Bell Pepper Stack with Basil Pesto

- **Snacks**: Baked Kale Chips with Nutritional Yeast (Appetizer), Tropical Immune Booster Smoothie with Pineapple, Mango, and Turmeric (Smoothie), Avocado Chocolate Mousse

(Dessert)

Day 5:

- **Breakfast**: Cottage Cheese with Pineapple Chunks and a Sprinkle of Chia Seeds

- **Lunch**: Grilled Chicken and Quinoa Salad with Avocado and Cucumber

- **Dinner**: Ginger Soy Glazed Salmon with Steamed Bok Choy and Brown Rice

- **Snacks**: Tomato and Basil Bruschetta on Whole Grain Bread (Appetizer), Peach and Oat Breakfast Smoothie (Smoothie), Almond and Date Energy Balls (Dessert)

Day 6:

- **Breakfast**: Buckwheat Pancakes with

Blueberry Compote

- **Lunch**: Roasted Vegetable and Chickpea Wrap with Hummus

- **Dinner**: Spinach and Feta Stuffed Chicken Breast with Quinoa Salad

- **Snacks**: Avocado and Shrimp Cocktail Cups (Appetizer), Carrot Cake Smoothie with Carrots, Walnuts, and Cinnamon (Smoothie), Coconut Yogurt with Fresh Mango and Toasted Coconut Flakes (Dessert)

Day 7:

- **Breakfast**: Quinoa Porridge with Almond Milk and Dried Apricots

- **Lunch**: Lentil and Spinach Stew with Brown Rice

- **Dinner**: Butternut Squash and Chickpea Curry with Brown Basmati Rice

- **Snacks**: Spinach and Feta Stuffed Mushrooms (Appetizer), Pomegranate and Beetroot Smoothie for Heart Health (Smoothie), Roasted Pear with Honey and Walnuts (Dessert)

Week 2:

Day 8:

- **Breakfast**: Scrambled Tofu with Kale and Tomatoes

- **Lunch**: Baked Salmon with Steamed Broccoli and Sweet Potato Mash

- **Dinner**: Zucchini Lasagna with Ricotta and Spinach

- **Snacks**: Sweet Potato and Black Bean Mini Tacos (Appetizer), Heart-Healthy Avocado and Cacao Smoothie (Smoothie), No-Bake Oatmeal and Peanut Butter Bars (Dessert)

Day 9:

- **Breakfast**: Muesli with Skimmed Milk, Sliced Pear, and Sunflower Seeds

- **Lunch**: Kale, Strawberry, and Walnut Salad with Grilled Tofu

- **Dinner**: Roasted Turmeric Cauliflower Steaks with Green Beans

- **Snacks**: Edamame and Mint Dip with Whole Wheat Pita Chips (Appetizer), Peach and Oat Breakfast Smoothie (Smoothie), Raspberry and Lemon Sorbet (Dessert)

Day 10:

- **Breakfast**: Baked Sweet Potato and Black Bean Breakfast Burritos

- **Lunch**: Spinach and Feta Stuffed Mushrooms

- **Dinner**: Portobello Mushroom Caps with Quinoa Pilaf and Steamed Kale

- **Snacks**: Grilled Asparagus Spears Wrapped in Prosciutto (Appetizer), Carrot Cake Smoothie with Carrots, Walnuts, and Cinnamon (Smoothie), Coconut Yogurt with Fresh Mango and Toasted Coconut Flakes (Dessert)

Day 11:

- **Breakfast**: Avocado and Egg Toast on Whole Grain Bread

- **Lunch**: Turmeric Cauliflower Soup with a side of Whole Grain Bread

- **Dinner**: Grilled Chicken and Quinoa Salad with Avocado and Cucumber

- **Snacks**: Cucumber and Hummus Bites

(Appetizer), Protein Power Smoothie with Almond Butter, Banana, and Hemp Seeds (Smoothie), Chia Seed Pudding with Mixed Berry Compote (Dessert)

Day 12:

- **Breakfast**: Greek Yogurt Parfait with Mixed Berries and Almonds

- **Lunch**: Zucchini Noodles with Pesto and Cherry Tomatoes

- **Dinner**: Moroccan Lentil and Sweet Potato Stew

- **Snacks**: Roasted Red Pepper and Walnut Dip with Whole Wheat Pita Chips (Appetizer), Green Detox Smoothie with Spinach, Kiwi, and Ginger (Smoothie), Baked Apples with Cinnamon and Nutmeg (Dessert)

Day 13:

- **Breakfast**: Oatmeal with Sliced Apple, Cinnamon, and Walnuts

- **Lunch**: Stuffed Bell Peppers with Quinoa, Black Beans, and Corn

- **Dinner**: Stuffed Acorn Squash with Wild Rice and Cranberries

- **Snacks**: Tomato and Basil Bruschetta on Whole Grain Bread (Appetizer), Berry Antioxidant Smoothie with Blueberries, Raspberries, and Flaxseed (Smoothie), Carrot and Walnut Muffins Sweetened with Apple Sauce (Dessert)

Day 14:

- **Breakfast**: Cottage Cheese with Pineapple Chunks and a Sprinkle of Chia Seeds

- **Lunch**: Grilled Chicken and Quinoa Salad with

Avocado and Cucumber

- **Dinner**: Ginger Soy Glazed Salmon with Steamed Bok Choy and Brown Rice

- **Snacks**: Zucchini and Carrot Fritters (Appetizer), Peach and Oat Breakfast Smoothie (Smoothie), Almond and Date Energy Balls (Dessert)

Week 3:

Day 15:

- **Breakfast**: Buckwheat Pancakes with Blueberry Compote

- **Lunch**: Roasted Vegetable and Chickpea Wrap with Hummus

- **Dinner**: Spinach and Feta Stuffed Chicken Breast with Quinoa Salad

- **Snacks**: Avocado and Shrimp Cocktail Cups

(Appetizer), Carrot Cake Smoothie with Carrots, Walnuts, and Cinnamon (Smoothie), Coconut Yogurt with Fresh Mango and Toasted Coconut Flakes (Dessert)

Day 16:

- **Breakfast**: Quinoa Porridge with Almond Milk and Dried Apricots

- **Lunch**: Lentil and Spinach Stew with Brown Rice

- **Dinner**: Butternut Squash and Chickpea Curry with Brown Basmati Rice

- **Snacks**: Spinach and Feta Stuffed Mushrooms (Appetizer), Pomegranate and Beetroot Smoothie for Heart Health (Smoothie), Roasted Pear with Honey and Walnuts (Dessert)

Day 17:

- **Breakfast**: Scrambled Tofu with Kale and Tomatoes

- **Lunch**: Baked Salmon with Steamed Broccoli and Sweet Potato Mash

- **Dinner**: Zucchini Lasagna with Ricotta and Spinach

- **Snacks**: Sweet Potato and Black Bean Mini Tacos (Appetizer), Heart-Healthy Avocado and Cacao Smoothie (Smoothie), No-Bake Oatmeal and Peanut Butter Bars (Dessert)

Day 18:

- **Breakfast**: Muesli with Skimmed Milk, Sliced Pear, and Sunflower Seeds

- **Lunch**: Kale, Strawberry, and Walnut Salad with Grilled Tofu

- **Dinner**: Roasted Turmeric Cauliflower Steaks

with Green Beans

- **Snacks**: Edamame and Mint Dip with Whole Wheat Pita Chips (Appetizer), Peach and Oat Breakfast Smoothie (Smoothie), Raspberry and Lemon Sorbet (Dessert)

Day 19:

- **Breakfast**: Baked Sweet Potato and Black Bean Breakfast Burritos

- **Lunch**: Spinach and Feta Stuffed Mushrooms

- **Dinner**: Portobello Mushroom Caps with Quinoa Pilaf and Steamed Kale

- **Snacks**: Grilled Asparagus Spears Wrapped in Prosciutto (Appetizer), Carrot Cake Smoothie with Carrots, Walnuts, and Cinnamon (Smoothie), Coconut Yogurt with Fresh Mango and Toasted Coconut Flakes (Dessert)

Day 20:

- **Breakfast**: Avocado and Egg Toast on Whole Grain Bread

- **Lunch**: Turmeric Cauliflower Soup with a side of Whole Grain Bread

- **Dinner**: Grilled Chicken and Quinoa Salad with Avocado and Cucumber

- **Snacks**: Cucumber and Hummus Bites (Appetizer), Protein Power Smoothie with Almond Butter, Banana, and Hemp Seeds (Smoothie), Chia Seed Pudding with Mixed Berry Compote (Dessert)

Day 21:

- **Breakfast**: Greek Yogurt Parfait with Mixed Berries and Almonds

- **Lunch:** Zucchini Noodles with Pesto and Cherry Tomatoes

- **Dinner**: Moroccan Lentil and Sweet Potato Stew

- **Snacks**: Roasted Red Pepper and Walnut Dip with Whole Wheat Pita Chips (Appetizer), Green Detox Smoothie with Spinach, Kiwi, and Ginger (Smoothie), Baked Apples with Cinnamon and Nutmeg (Dessert)

Week 4

Day 22:

- **Breakfast**: Oatmeal with Sliced Apple, Cinnamon, and Walnuts

- **Lunch**: Stuffed Bell Peppers with Quinoa, Black Beans, and Corn

- **Dinner**: Stuffed Acorn Squash with Wild Rice and Cranberries

- **Snacks**: Tomato and Basil Bruschetta on Whole Grain Bread (Appetizer), Berry Antioxidant Smoothie with Blueberries, Raspberries, and Flaxseed (Smoothie), Carrot and Walnut Muffins Sweetened with Apple Sauce (Dessert)

Day 23:

- **Breakfast**: Cottage Cheese with Pineapple Chunks and a Sprinkle of Chia Seeds

- **Lunch**: Grilled Chicken and Quinoa Salad with Avocado and Cucumber

- **Dinner**: Ginger Soy Glazed Salmon with Steamed Bok Choy and Brown Rice

- **Snacks**: Zucchini and Carrot Fritters (Appetizer), Peach and Oat Breakfast Smoothie (Smoothie), Almond and Date Energy Balls (Dessert)

Day 24:

- **Breakfast**: Buckwheat Pancakes with Blueberry Compote

- **Lunch**: Roasted Vegetable and Chickpea Wrap with Hummus

- **Dinner**: Spinach and Feta Stuffed Chicken Breast with Quinoa Salad

- **Snacks**: Avocado and Shrimp Cocktail Cups (Appetizer), Carrot Cake Smoothie with Carrots, Walnuts, and Cinnamon (Smoothie), Coconut Yogurt with Fresh Mango and Toasted Coconut Flakes (Dessert)

Day 25:

- **Breakfast**: Quinoa Porridge with Almond Milk and Dried Apricots

- **Lunch**: Lentil and Spinach Stew with Brown Rice

- **Dinner**: Butternut Squash and Chickpea Curry with Brown Basmati Rice

- **Snacks**: Spinach and Feta Stuffed Mushrooms (Appetizer), Pomegranate and Beetroot Smoothie for Heart Health (Smoothie), Roasted Pear with Honey and Walnuts (Dessert)

Day 26:

- **Breakfast**: Scrambled Tofu with Kale and Tomatoes

- **Lunch**: Baked Salmon with Steamed Broccoli and Sweet Potato Mash

- **Dinner**: Zucchini Lasagna with Ricotta and Spinach

- **Snacks**: Sweet Potato and Black Bean Mini Tacos (Appetizer), Heart-Healthy Avocado and

Cacao Smoothie (Smoothie), No-Bake Oatmeal and Peanut Butter Bars (Dessert)

Day 27:

- **Breakfast**: Muesli with Skimmed Milk, Sliced Pear, and Sunflower Seeds

- **Lunch**: Kale, Strawberry, and Walnut Salad with Grilled Tofu

- **Dinner**: Roasted Turmeric Cauliflower Steaks with Green Beans

- **Snacks**: Edamame and Mint Dip with Whole Wheat Pita Chips (Appetizer), Peach and Oat Breakfast Smoothie (Smoothie), Raspberry and Lemon Sorbet (Dessert)

Day 28:

- **Breakfast**: Baked Sweet Potato and Black Bean Breakfast Burritos

- **Lunch**: Spinach and Feta Stuffed Mushrooms

- **Dinner**: Portobello Mushroom Caps with Quinoa Pilaf and Steamed Kale

- **Snacks**: Grilled Asparagus Spears Wrapped in Prosciutto (Appetizer), Carrot Cake Smoothie with Carrots, Walnuts, and Cinnamon (Smoothie), Coconut Yogurt with Fresh Mango and Toasted Coconut Flakes (Dessert)

Day 29:

- **Breakfast**: Avocado and Egg Toast on Whole Grain Bread

- **Lunch**: Turmeric Cauliflower Soup with a side of Whole Grain Bread

- **Dinner**: Grilled Chicken and Quinoa Salad with

Avocado and Cucumber

- **Snacks**: Cucumber and Hummus Bites (Appetizer), Protein Power Smoothie with Almond Butter, Banana, and Hemp Seeds (Smoothie), Chia Seed Pudding with Mixed Berry Compote (Dessert)

Day 30:

- **Breakfast**: Greek Yogurt Parfait with Mixed Berries and Almonds

- **Lunch**: Zucchini Noodles with Pesto and Cherry Tomatoes

- **Dinner**: Moroccan Lentil and Sweet Potato Stew

- **Snacks**: Roasted Red Pepper and Walnut Dip with Whole Wheat Pita Chips (Appetizer), Green Detox Smoothie with Spinach, Kiwi, and Ginger (Smoothie), Baked Apples with Cinnamon and

Nutmeg (Dessert)

FOOD DIARY

TIME	MEALS	FOOD AND DRINK CONSUMED	MOOD	CRAVING	ENERGY LEVEL	SLEEP QUALITY

FOOD DIARY

TIME	MEALS	FOOD AND DRINK CONSUMED	MOOD	CRAVING	ENERGY LEVEL	SLEEP QUALITY

FOOD DIARY

TIME	MEALS	FOOD AND DRINK CONSUMED	MOOD	CRAVING	ENERGY LEVEL	SLEEP QUALITY

FOOD DIARY

TIME	MEALS	FOOD AND DRINK CONSUMED	MOOD	CRAVING	ENERGY LEVEL	SLEEP QUALITY

FOOD DIARY

TIME	MEALS	FOOD AND DRINK CONSUMED	MOOD	CRAVING	ENERGY LEVEL	SLEEP QUALITY

FOOD DIARY

TIME	MEALS	FOOD AND DRINK CONSUMED	MOOD	CRAVING	ENERGY LEVEL	SLEEP QUALITY

FOOD DIARY

TIME	MEALS	FOOD AND DRINK CONSUMED	MOOD	CRAVING	ENERGY LEVEL	SLEEP QUALITY

FOOD DIARY

TIME	MEALS	FOOD AND DRINK CONSUMED	MOOD	CRAVING	ENERGY LEVEL	SLEEP QUALITY

FOOD DIARY

TIME	MEALS	FOOD AND DRINK CONSUMED	MOOD	CRAVING	ENERGY LEVEL	SLEEP QUALITY

FOOD DIARY

TIME	MEALS	FOOD AND DRINK CONSUMED	MOOD	CRAVING	ENERGY LEVEL	SLEEP QUALITY

FOOD DIARY

TIME	MEALS	FOOD AND DRINK CONSUMED	MOOD	CRAVING	ENERGY LEVEL	SLEEP QUALITY

FOOD DIARY

TIME	MEALS	FOOD AND DRINK CONSUMED	MOOD	CRAVING	ENERGY LEVEL	SLEEP QUALITY

FOOD DIARY

TIME	MEALS	FOOD AND DRINK CONSUMED	MOOD	CRAVING	ENERGY LEVEL	SLEEP QUALITY

FOOD DIARY

TIME	MEALS	FOOD AND DRINK CONSUMED	MOOD	CRAVING	ENERGY LEVEL	SLEEP QUALITY

FOOD DIARY

TIME	MEALS	FOOD AND DRINK CONSUMED	MOOD	CRAVING	ENERGY LEVEL	SLEEP QUALITY

THANK YOU FOR CHOOSING "THE BREAST CANCER DIET COOKBOOK FOR WOMEN OVER 50"

By choosing this cookbook, you've taken a significant step towards embracing a healthier, more joyful journey in the face of breast cancer. It takes courage to face breast cancer head-on, and even more to make lifestyle changes that support your health and well-being during this time. Each page you turn, every recipe you try, is a testament to your strength and determination. I am honored to be a part of your journey, providing not just meals, but moments of joy, comfort, and empowerment.

Every recipe in this book was crafted with love, care, and a deep understanding of the unique challenges and needs faced by women over 50 battling breast cancer. I believe that food is more than just sustenance; it's a source of comfort, a means of healing, and a celebration of life itself. By bringing these recipes into your kitchen, you're inviting a world of flavor, health, and healing.

I'd love to hear from you. Your feedback, stories, and insights are invaluable, helping me to make this resource even better for women just like you. Please don't hesitate to reach out, share your journey, or ask questions. Together, we can continue to make a difference.

Thank you for allowing me to be a part of your healing journey. May each recipe bring you not just nutritional benefits but also moments of happiness, a sense of achievement, and a celebration of the vibrant life you lead.

Here's to your health, your resilience, and your journey.

Warmest regards,

Elizabeth V. Carrington

www.ingramcontent.com/pod-product-compliance
Lightning Source LLC
Chambersburg PA
CBHW050803260726
48660CB00004B/1217